Learning from
Health Action Zones

Learning from
Health Action Zones

Edited by

Dr. Linda Bauld & Professor Ken Judge
University of Glasgow, Scotland

Aeneas

First published in 2002
by Aeneas Press

PO Box 200
Chichester
West Sussex
PO18 OYX
UK

Typeset in AGaramond
by Marie Doherty

Printed and bound by
MPG Books
Victoria Square
Bodmin
Cornwall
UK

ISBN: 1-902115-24-4

British Library Cataloguing in Publication Data
A catalogue record of this book is available from the British Library

Bauld, Linda & Judge, Ken

Acknowledgements

The national evaluation of Health Action Zones is funded by the Department of Health. The views expressed in the introduction, conclusion and forewords in this book are those of the authors and not necessarily those of the Department of Health.

The editors would like to thank the following individuals for their support: Julie Truman, who organised the local/national evaluation conference that served as the starting point for this book; Lee Adams, Graham Brown and colleagues from Wakefield Health Action Zone who hosted the conference; Anand Kumar from Aeneas Ltd; and Amitti Canaga Retna and members of the HAZ central team in the Department of Health. We would also like to acknowledge the contribution of Merle Read, who copy-edited the book, and Martha McCorkindale, who provided administrative support.

List of contributors

Lee Adams, Director, Wakefield Health Action Zone

Pete Alcock, Professor of Social Policy and Administration, University of Birmingham

Sheena Asthana, Principal Lecturer/Director of HAZ Evaluation Programme, Department of Social Policy and Social Work, University of Plymouth

Marian Barnes, Director of Social Research, Department of Social Policy & Social Work, University of Birmingham

Linda Bauld, Lecturer in Social Policy, Department of Social Policy & Social Work, University of Glasgow

Jean Bell, Centre Manager, Briardale Community and Training Centre, Blyth

Michaela Benzeval, Senior Lecturer, Health Research Group, Department of Geography, Queen Mary University of London

Sohail Bhatti, Consultant in Public Health Medicine, Wirral Health Authority (now Public Health Lead for West Lancashire Primary Care NHS Trust, Ormskirk)

Janet Bostock, Clinical Community Psychologist, Northumberland Health Action Zone/Northumberland Mental Health Trust

Graham Brown, Policy and Research Co-ordinator, Wakefield Health Action Zone

Judith Brown, Community Enterprise Advisor, Northumberland County Council, Bomarsund

Robin Bunton, Reader in Social Policy, School of Social Sciences and Law, University of Teesside

Salma Burton, Health Action Zone Evaluation and Research Manager, Camden and Islington Health Authority

Ben Cave, East London and the City Health Action Zone and Renaisi, and Visiting Research Fellow, Health Research Group, Department of Geography, Queen Mary University of London

Michael Clark, Research and Development Co-ordinator, Wolverhampton Health Care NHS Trust

Dara Coppel, Evaluation, Learning and Development Manager, Nottingham City Primary Care Trust

Lesley Cotterill, Senior Lecturer/Evaluation Advisor, Department of Sociology, University of Plymouth

Gary Craig, Professor of Social Justice, Department of Comparative and Applied Social Sciences, University of Hull.

Paul Crawshaw, Lecturer in Research Methods, School of Health and Social Care, University of Teesside

Sarah Curtis, Professor of Health Geography, Health Research Group, Department of Geography, Queen Mary University of London

Veronica Cuthbert, Public Health Facilitator, Birkenhead Primary Care Group (formerly Health Visitor with Wirral & West Cheshire Community NHS Trust)

Chris Dabbs, Co-ordinator, School for Social Entrepreneurs, and Chief Officer, Salford Community Health Council

David Diaz de Leon, University of Texas Health Science Center, Houston, USA

Anna Downie, Evaluation Officer, Leeds Health Action Zone

Eleanor Green, Assistant Director, Health Promotion Strategy, Bradford Health Authority

Kate Gillen, Principal Lecturer in Psychology, Business School, University of Sunderland

Joyce Halliday, Senior Research Fellow/HAZ Evaluation Programme Manager, Department of Social Policy and Social Work, University of Plymouth

Claire Holden, Evaluation and Research Manager, Sheffield Health Action Zone

Sue Holden, Research Associate, Department of Public Health and Primary Care, University of Hull

Brian Jacobs, Professor, Centre for Health Policy and Practice, Staffordshire University

Ken Judge, Professor, HEBS Chair of Health Promotion Policy, Department of Public Health, University of Glasgow

Brigid Kane, South Yorkshire Coalfields Health Action Zone Co-ordinator

Louise Lawson, Research Associate, Health Promotion Policy Unit, Department of Public Health, University of Glasgow

Jane Lunt, Public Health Facilitator, Birkenhead Primary Care Group (formerly Health Visitor with Wirral & West Cheshire Community NHS Trust)

Mhairi Mackenzie, Research Fellow, Health Promotion Policy Unit, Department of Public Health, University of Glasgow

Jane Mackinnon, Research Associate, Health Promotion Policy Unit, Department of Social Policy, University of Glasgow

Elizabeth Matka, Research Fellow, Department of Social Policy & Social Work, University of Birmingham

Fiona Meth, Research Officer, Health Research Group, Department of Geography, Queen Mary University of London

Susan Mulroy, Centre for Health Policy and Practice, Staffordshire University

Rachel Munton, Senior Education Co-ordinator, Leicester City Health Action Zone (now Director of Mental Health Nursing, Department of Health)

Madeleine J. Murtagh, Department of Epidemiology and Public Health, University of Newcastle Upon Tyne, and Northern and Yorkshire Public Health Observatory

Sian Penner, Regeneration & Employment Workstream Manager, City & East London Health Action Zone

Sue Richardson, Research Fellow, Department of Social Policy and Social Work, University of Plymouth

Liz Rodrigo, Education Co-ordinator, Leicester City Health Action Zone

Christine Sime, Centre for Health Policy and Practice, Staffordshire University

Jane Sharpe, Assistant Psychologist, Northumberland Health Action Zone/Northumberland Mental Health Trust

Jane South, Researcher, Health Action Zone Evaluation, Department of Applied Social Sciences, University of Bradford

Jane Springett, Professor of Health Promotion and Public Health, Institute for Health, Liverpool John Moores University

Sandra Squires, Senior Evaluator, Wolverhampton HAZ

Michael Stores, Head of Information Services, Let's Get Serious Ltd

Richard Strittmatter, Managing Director, Let's Get Serious Ltd

Helen Sullivan, Lecturer in Local Government Policy, School of Public Policy, Institute of Local Government Studies, University of Birmingham

Angela Young, Senior Research Fellow, Institute for Public Health Research & Policy, University of Salford

Contents

The development of Health Action Zones

Linda Bauld and Ken Judge

Health Action Zones were established early in the life of a new government committed to improving population health and tackling inequalities across the UK. HAZs were the first area-based initiative to be established by New Labour and were intended to be 'trailblazers' for new ways of working between the NHS and other agencies to address long-standing health problems in England's most deprived communities.

The idea of HAZs was originally announced by Frank Dobson, the then Secretary of State for Health, in June 1997. He described them as pilot projects 'to explore mechanisms for breaking through current organisational boundaries to tackle inequalities, and deliver better services and better health care, building upon and encouraging co-operation across the NHS' (DoH, 1997). In October 1997 health authorities in conjunction with local authorities and other agencies were invited to submit bids to become Health Action Zones. In the call for bids, the three strategic objectives of HAZs were as follows (DoH, 1997):

- to identify and address the public health needs of the local area
- to increase the effectiveness, efficiency and responsiveness of services
- to develop partnerships for improving people's health and relevant services, adding value through creating synergy between the work of different agencies.

Among the benefits offered to potential HAZs were new freedoms, flexibilities and resources, although these were not spelled out in great detail. HAZs were intended to have a lifespan of up to seven years, providing an opportunity to invest in sustainable change. They would be supported by a central policy team based at the NHS Executive in Leeds. In return each HAZ was expected to establish partnership boards; to demonstrate community involvement; to set targets for potential achievements, including early wins; invest in local evaluation; and to set in place performance management systems that would monitor and demonstrate progress with reference to agreed milestones (HAZ National Evaluation Team, 1999).

Forty-one bids for Health Action Zone status were received by the DoH from 49 health authorities. From these, Health Action Zone status was awarded to 11 areas from April 1998. Of those areas not selected in the first wave, a number were asked to submit further applications (along with other areas of high deprivation), and 15 more were granted HAZ status from April 1999. Those health authorities that were successful in gaining HAZ status were provided with additional resources – although these were fairly modest, a collective allocation of £320 million over three years (1998/99–2001/02), representing less than 1% of NHS resources. This included earmarked funds for drugs prevention projects, smoking cessation services, innovation projects and employment and health projects. In addition, HAZs would receive some money for development support, amounting to approximately £100,000 per year per HAZ.

Background

HAZs are complex entities that vary considerably in their size, history and way of working. At their heart, they are partnerships that involve a range of local agencies in specific health improvement activities. Most HAZs have a core team of support staff (led by a project manager/director) who work with a partnership board made up of representatives from health and local authorities, other public sector organisations (such as the police and universities), the voluntary sector, private sector and community groups. Through this partnership structure, HAZs have used the funds allocated to them by central government and resources from local agencies to invest in a wide range of different types of projects and activities.

In total, HAZ areas cover 13 million people in England, representing over a third of the total population (see Figure 1). The smallest HAZ contains approximately 200,000 people and the largest more than 1.4 million. The geographical and organisational configuration of HAZs falls into four categories:

- multiple health authority, multiple local authority – such as Merseyside and Tyne and Wear
- single health authority, multiple local authority – such as Nottingham and Camden and Islington
- co-terminous health and local authority – including Bradford, Sandwell, Wakefield and others
- sub-health-authority and local authority – such as Plymouth and Luton.

HAZs also cover both urban and rural areas, with some HAZs (such as Hull and East Riding) containing a mix of both. Other local factors, such as the

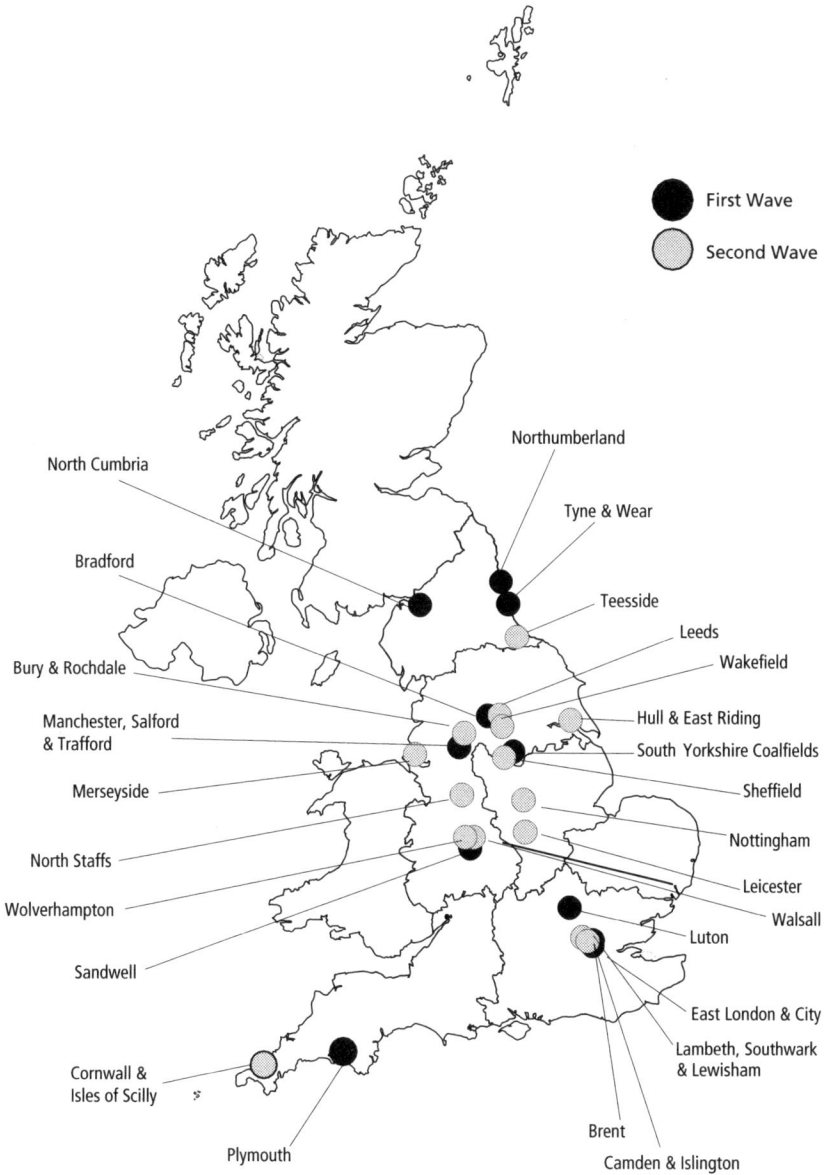

Figure 1: Health Action Zones in England

extent and history of partnership working between agencies, patterns of employment in the area and ethnic diversity, also vary considerably between HAZs.

What all these areas share, however, is a common history of deprivation and poor health. Using the DETR index of deprivation (DETR, 2000), 81 of the most 100 deprived wards in England are located within Health Action Zones. In addition, half of all HAZ wards are in the most deprived quintile of wards in England as a whole, and less that 20 per cent of all HAZ wards are in the 50 per cent least deprived wards in the country (Adams et al., 2000). In relation to poor health, earlier work we have done suggests that, using key indicators from the Health Survey of England and ONS vital statistics for health authorities, HAZ areas have significantly higher levels of poor health than other parts of the country (HAZ National Evaluation Team, 1999). There is a strong correlation between the degree of deprivation in each HAZ and the level of poor health.

The diversity of HAZs is demonstrated not only through variations in areas, organisational complexity, population coverage and profile, but also in the wide range of projects and activities that they have invested in. To a certain degree, these activities have varied through time as policy changes have affected the development of HAZs, a point we return to below. However, it is possible to describe the range of HAZ projects and programmes, and provide some examples.

Initial analysis of the first HAZ plans produced by all 26 zones revealed over 200 separate programmes of work, and within those, over 2000 separate projects or activities. A broad categorisation of programmes revealed seven main types, focusing on:

- population groups (such as older people, black and ethnic minority groups)
- health problems (such as cancer, mental health)
- root causes of ill health (e.g. housing, employment, lifestyle issues)
- health and social care (health promotion, acute care)
- community empowerment
- internal processes (such as strategy development, local evaluation)
- a combination of these.

Following this initial analysis, a key source of information regarding the range of HAZ activities has been the quarterly performance management reports that HAZs submit to the Department of Health. One component of these reports is 'high level statement' documentation, which describes HAZ projects in a structured format and outlines progress made towards targets and milestones. An analysis of the June 2000 documentation identified 264 high level statements, ranging from 3 to 36 per HAZ, with a mean of 10 (Bauld et al., 2001). Sheffield, for instance, provided 3 high level statements that were very broad-ranging, encompassing numerous projects within each. These were: disease management, promoting independence, and root causes. Teesside, on the other hand, adopted an area-based approach and provided 36 high level statements. It has developed separate programmes of activity for specific areas within Teesside (Middlesbrough, Hartlepool, Stockton, Redcar and Cleveland) around the key themes of improving health (lifestyles, environment), smoking cessation, teenage pregnancy, young people's lifestyles, caring for vulnerable people, saving lives and modernising strategies.

Within this wide range of activity, it is possible to identify common approaches to health improvement. In aiming to address the needs of a particular population group, for instance, HAZs can invest in activities that have a clinical focus or a behavioural focus, or indeed aim to improve community or environmental conditions. Table 1 provides examples from HAZ high level statements that focus on children and young people.

Since they were established HAZs have been at the forefront of attempts to modernise health services and to reduce health inequalities. As a result there is much to learn from the efforts they have made. But the path that HAZs have taken, and the learning that they have generated, is not a straightforward one.

Table 1 Children and young people: examples of HAZ activities/programmes

Clinical focus	Behavioural focus	Structural/environmental focus
• Asthma prevention and treatment	• Teenage pregnancy	• Healthy schools
• Specialist child health services, e.g. paediatric cardiology	• Sexual health	• Work with looked-after children, children at risk, young people leaving care
• Speech therapy services	• Healthy schools (behaviour focus)	• Links with Sure Start and Sure Start Plus
• Low birth-weight babies	• Lifestyles – healthy eating, exercise	• Links with Education Action Zones
• Immunisation	• Sun-safety projects	• Food initiatives – breakfast clubs, food co-ops
• Children with complex medical needs	• Smoking cessation	• Rent deposit scheme
	• Mental health interventions	• Mental health interventions
	• Breastfeeding	• Youth crime
	• Oral health	• Including children and young people in planning and service delivery/youth forums
	• Drug work, substance misuse	• Links with Single Regeneration Budget
	• Youth crime	• Links with Home Start
	• Proof-of-age scheme	• Links with New Deal for Communities
	• Reducing accidents	
	• Bullying work	

The past three years have seen an enormous amount of institutional and policy turbulence associated with the NHS and local government in England. New initiatives and changes in policy emphasis have emerged from Whitehall on an almost continuous basis, and this has sometimes made it hard to maintain the commitment of all parties at the local level to a sustainable strategy and deliver health change. Fortunately there are now signs that a greater degree of organisational stability is likely. If this occurs then there will be many opportunities for HAZs to contribute to the strengthening of local public health strategies.

The main purpose of this book is to provide some practical illustrations of the types of learning that are available. But before we introduce some features of the approach to learning adopted in relation to HAZs, it is important to provide a brief indication of some of the challenges they have faced.

Challenges

Despite the complexity and diversity of HAZs, they have been subject to a common set of evolving national policy priorities since their establishment. Changes in policy direction have combined with local circumstances to result in a difficult process of development for HAZs.

Particular challenges have included:

- partnerships and planning mechanisms
- performance management
- changing policy priorities.

For many HAZs, it took time to put partnership arrangements in place. Historical differences between organisations were a problem in some areas. In one HAZ, for instance, relevant district councils became closely involved, but the engagement of the county council was limited. In another HAZ, one of three local authorities in the area initially became involved but later withdrew much of its support. In many HAZs the process of engaging the voluntary sector and community groups proved difficult. What most HAZs discovered was that both building and sustaining complex partnerships takes time and continued effort (Barnes et al., 2001).

An additional challenge for HAZs, particularly in the early stages of their development, involves their capacity to plan and implement projects and programmes. Our early work identified a credibility gap between the longer-term aspirations of HAZs and the projects they had chosen to invest in (Judge, 2000). HAZ partners were able to identify the problems in their local community that they wished to address, and what they wanted to achieve in terms of health improvement and tackling inequalities. But articulating how specific activities would achieve particular intermediate outcomes that would in turn contribute to the realisation of final goals proved extremely difficult. To some extent this is an ongoing problem for HAZs. This limited local capacity to develop robust and convincing plans has in some cases seriously inhibited the potential for learning.

One response to planning problems from the Department of Health has been the development of a distinct performance management framework for HAZs. This framework has been accompanied by varied forms of investment in central support (such as workshops for project managers regarding the use of project planning tools, for example 'logframe' approaches). As we have already mentioned, HAZs are expected to submit quarterly high level statement and other documentation to the DoH both to demonstrate how resources are being used and to provide evidence of progress towards their objectives. While this type of central monitoring does promote accountability, the development and initial implementation of the HAZ performance management framework were not without their problems. It has been perceived as a straightjacket by many HAZs, and symptomatic of New Labour's emphasis on central control and target setting. In interviews with project managers in 2000, we specifically sought views regarding performance management. Many project managers reported that high level statement documentation neither represented a true reflection of their work nor helped to deliver real change on the ground. As one HAZ project manager explained at the time (Bauld et al., 2001): 'The high level statement doesn't really give us what we need locally, or the same sort of format that we've been developing in our plans. It is a pain to have to produce something in a format which we don't feel is useful.'

An additional centrally imposed challenge for HAZs has been shifting national policy priorities. HAZs were initially given considerable local discretion to select priority areas for action, and the result was that the original plans for both first- and second-wave zones addressed a very wide range of issues. As a senior civil servant involved in the early stages of implementation told us: 'We felt very much that this was a bottom-up initiative, whose partners were not just the NHS but local authorities and other local organisations. We intended all local partners to agree a challenging programme for themselves that met their identified health and health care needs.'

However, New Labour's plans for wider NHS reform, particularly those conceived by the new Secretary of State, Alan Milburn (who replaced Frank Dobson early in 2000), were not particularly compatible with this locally determined agenda. The result was increasing pressure on HAZs to modify existing programmes to contribute to the achievement of overall NHS objectives, such as tackling waiting lists and addressing cancer, coronary heart disease and mental health issues.

The difficulties that HAZs experienced in planning their activities and developing partnerships contributed to other problems in 2000. The initial enthusiasm that HAZs had engendered at the local and national level began to wane, and in some HAZs slow development contributed to an underspend in relation to particular projects and programmes. The result was cuts to core HAZ budgets. This combined with the growing realisation, following the publication of the NHS Plan in June 2000, that HAZs were unlikely to continue in their current form for the seven-year lifespan they had been promised.

Thus Health Action Zones have experienced considerable turbulence since the establishment of the first wave of zones in 1998. This brief overview of the national context is important, as the research reported in this book was largely conducted during these early stages of HAZ development. What is important to emphasise, however, is that the policy context for HAZs in 2002 has again changed and looks much more positive. The concluding chapter in this volume reviews some of these recent changes and reflects on the important contribution that HAZs can make to emerging structures, such as local strategic partnerships and primary care groups.

Learning

Learning from HAZs was intended from the beginning, with 'taking an evidence-based approach' included as one of the seven underpinning principles of the initiative. In addition, the Department of Health commissioned a national evaluation early in the lifetime of HAZs and emphasised the importance of local evaluation efforts. Since then, the turbulent policy environment surrounding HAZs and the challenges they have faced in planning and implementing their activities have meant that evaluation has been undertaken in difficult circumstances. But learning from HAZs remains of central importance. This book is a joint effort between members of the national evaluation team and local evaluators. Before describing its origins and content, it is worth briefly describing the main components of the national evaluation and links with local evaluation efforts.

National evaluation

In the spring of 1998, at the same time as the first wave of Health Action Zones was being selected, the Department of Health invited applications to undertake the central or national evaluation of HAZs. The centrally commissioned evaluation was intended 'to address strategic issues of importance for central policy on Health Action Zones and the wider policy agenda of the NHS White Paper and the Green Paper "Our Healthier Nation" … [and] to contribute valuable lessons to support HAZ development locally' (DoH, 1998).

The research brief highlighted the fact that Health Action Zones are expected to have a life of five to seven years and that the central evaluation 'will need to be capable of assessing interim achievements as well as longer term impact'. Beyond this the DoH recognised the very wide scope of what HAZs might try to do. Even so it was expected that 'the evaluation should be concerned with assessing processes as well as outcomes and impact, to ascertain how as well as whether objectives are achieved'.

Given the uncertainty about the development of the HAZ initiative and the type of national evaluation that was required, the commissioning process was considerably protracted, and it was not until the end of 1998 that a contract was agreed for a modest first phase of national evaluation. The initial contract was for two years. Following the submission of a scoping report in June 1999 (HAZ National Evaluation Team, 1999) and further negotiations regarding evaluation design, the research contract was extended to the end of 2002.

The overarching aim of the national evaluation is to identify and assess the conditions in which strategies to create a more substantial *capacity for local collaboration* result in the adoption of *change mechanisms* that lead to the *modernisation of services* and a *reduction in health inequalities*.

This aim is being tackled in two distinct ways: through the monitoring and mapping of all 26 HAZs, and through a more detailed investigation of the change process in a selection of HAZs. The work is being conducted by researchers based at the University of Glasgow, the University of Birmingham and Queen Mary, University of London. Figure 2 overleaf outlines the main components of the study design.

The monitoring (undertaken by the members of the Glasgow team) provides a basic description of overall change strategies, the way in which these develop and the progress that is made by HAZs within the three years of the evaluation.

In contrast three separate groupings of case studies have been developed to allow for more detailed interrogation of the key evaluation questions:

• The University of Glasgow is investigating eight integrated case-study sites. Within these case studies the aim is to gain an understanding of the process of change at a strategic level, including a focus on visions and goals, and measuring progress.
• The University of Birmingham is progressing the component of the evaluation that focuses on HAZ strategies for building capacity for collaboration within five case studies.
• Responsibility for the third element of the evaluation (specific interventions aimed at tackling inequalities) rests with members of the evaluation team at

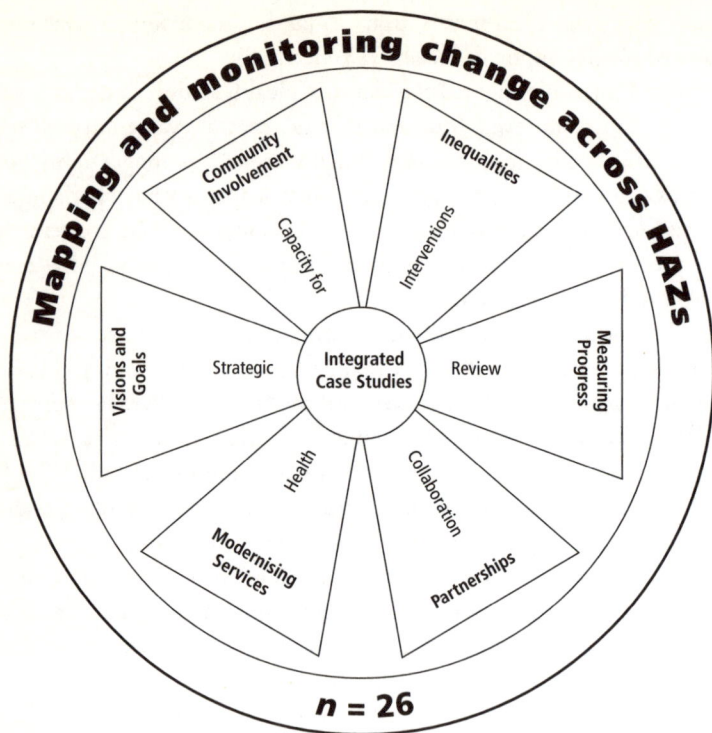

Figure 2: National Evaluation Framework

Queen Mary, University of London, who are conducting this work in three HAZ case study areas. Queen Mary researchers are also contributing to the integrated case study work.

What links the different components of the research is a common approach to evaluation. An approach should be recognised as distinct from research methods, as it can encompass multiple methods. Indeed, a variety of both quantitative and qualitative methodologies is being used to evaluate HAZs. But what we have found is that the investigation of an initiative as complex as HAZs – where activities and their outcomes are intimately associated with a changing policy environment and shifting local circumstances – does not easily lend itself to traditional evaluation.

Our approach is drawn primarily from two frameworks for evaluation that were developed to guide the assessment of social programmes operating in complex open systems such as disadvantaged communities. The first approach has been widely used in the UK in Home Office research, and is called *realistic evaluation* (Pawson and Tilley, 1997). The second is a *theories of change* approach to evaluation, which is well established in North America (Connell et al., 1995). Together, they provide a *theory-based approach* to the evaluation of the community health improvement process in HAZs (Judge and Bauld, 2001). More details regarding the approach and its components can be found in the foreword to Section 2.

Local evaluation

In addition to the national research, individual HAZs have also invested in evaluation. The strategies adopted have varied across the 26 areas. Some HAZs have invested considerable resources in evaluation, while others have placed less emphasis on local learning and more on delivery. An in-depth investigation of local learning approaches in the eight integrated case-study sites for the national evaluation has recently been completed, and provides some useful examples (Lawson et al., 2002).

The most common approach to local evaluation has been to employ an evaluation manager (either directly or through a university contract), but the precise role of the individual varies, from collecting project management data to being actively engaged in providing individual projects and programmes with the support to conduct self-evaluation, in many cases using theory-based approaches.

Other HAZs have established a strategic level evaluation group and evaluation teams or managers who focus on specific types of HAZ activity. In South Yorkshire Coalfields, for example, each of the HAZ's three work programme areas has an evaluation team associated with it. Within the Children and Young People programme there is a full-time evaluation officer who provides support to individual projects; for the Disability in Later Life programme, evaluation is contracted out to an academic unit; and for Heart Health there is a development officer who works in conjunction with an academic unit to produce an overall programme evaluation (Lawson et al., 2002).

Finally, a small number of HAZs have invested in evaluation programmes conducted entirely by an external university team. In some cases these evaluations have focused on progress across the HAZ as a whole, and in other instances they have examined specific projects for a specified period of time.

The range and diversity of local evaluation approaches means that there is a considerable amount of evidence emerging regarding HAZ activities. Since 1998 a key mechanism for sharing some of this learning has been the local/national HAZ evaluation network. This network began to meet informally through the efforts of local evaluators in Luton HAZ and others. The national evaluation team was involved from the beginning, and subsequent discussions with the

Department of Health resulted in a coordination and synthesis role being included in the national evaluation research design. As a result, the national team has been responsible for maintaining the network since 1999.

The HAZ local/national evaluation network communicates via an email discussion list managed by the HAZnet team based at the Health Development Agency in London. In addition, regular meetings of the network are held twice a year. These involve a full day of paper presentations and discussions. This book draws on papers presented at the local/national evaluation network meeting hosted by Wakefield and District HAZ on 7 September 2001.

Structure of the book

The Wakefield conference was organised around three themes of ongoing importance to Health Action Zones: capacity for collaboration (which focuses on engaging communities and partnership working), learning (examining local evaluation methods/findings and other forms of local learning) and innovation (examining progressive projects and programmes in HAZs). This book adopts the same structure, and includes contributors to the conference as well as a number of other local evaluators.

An overview to each section is provided by the three forewords, each written by members of the national evaluation team. The first is by Helen Sullivan, Marian Barnes and Elizabeth Matka, who are based at the University of Birmingham. Their research has focused on HAZ efforts to involve communities and build effective partnerships. The foreword they have written summarises key findings from their work with five Health Action Zones, and introduces each of the chapters in the 'building capacity for collaboration' section. The second foreword is by Mhairi Mackenzie, Louise Lawson and Jane Mackinnon, members of the evaluation team based at Glasgow University. They describe the role of HAZs as learning organisations, outline a theory-based approach to evaluation and introduce the contributions from local evaluators that make up the 'generating learning' section of the book. Finally, Michaela Benzeval and Fiona Meth from Queen Mary College at the University of London introduce the 'innovation' chapters. They reflect on the HAZ objective of reducing health inequalities and investing in innovative approaches to health improvement, before summarising key components of each of the chapters in the innovations section. The book concludes with a short chapter that looks to the future of Health Action Zones, and reflects on the potential learning they have to offer other complex community initiatives.

References

Adams, C., Bauld, L. and Judge, K. (2000) *Leading the way: smoking cessation services in Health Action Zones*, Glasgow: University of Glasgow, Health Promotion Policy Unit [available at http://www.haznet.org.uk/hazs/evidence/leading-the-wayDec2000.pdf]

Barnes, M., Sullivan, H. and Matka, E. (2001) *Building capacity for collaboration: the national evaluation of Health Action Zones, context, strategy and capacity: initial findings from the strategic level analysis, HAZ strategic overview report*, Birmingham: University of Birmingham [available at http://www.haznet.org.uk/hazs/evidence/nat_evalCIJul2001.pdf].

Bauld, L., Judge, K., Lawson, L., Mackenzie, M., Mackinnon, J. and Truman, J. (2001) *Health Action Zones in transition: progress in 2000*, Glasgow: University of Glasgow, Health Promotion Policy Unit [available from: http://www.haznet.org.uk/hazs/evidence/nat_evalrptMay01.pdf].

Connell, J. P., Kubisch, A.C., Schorr, L.B. and Weiss, C.H. (eds) (1995) *New approaches to evaluating community initiatives: concepts, methods and contexts*, Washington, DC: The Aspen Institute.

DETR (2000) *Index of multiple deprivation*, London: The Stationery Office/Department of the Environment, Transport and the Regions.

DoH (1997) *Health Action Zones: invitation to bid*, EL (97) 65, 30 October, Leeds: Department of Health.

DoH (1998) *National evaluation of Health Action Zones: call for research proposals*, London: Department of Health.

HAZ National Evaluation Team (1999) *Health Action Zones: learning to make a difference. Findings from a preliminary review of Health Action Zones and proposals for a national evaluation: a report submitted to the Department of Health*, PSSRU Discussion Paper 1546, June, Canterbury: University of Kent at Canterbury [available at http://www.ukc.ac.uk/PSSRU/downloads/ddp1546.html].

Judge, K (2000) 'Testing evaluation to the limits: the case of English Health Action Zones', *Journal of Health Services Research and Policy*, 5/1, 3–6.

Judge, K. and Bauld, L. (2001) 'Strong theory, flexible methods: evaluating complex community-based initiatives', *Critical Public Health*, 11/1, 19–38.

Lawson, L., Mackenzie, M., Mackinnon, J, Meth, F. and Truman, J. (2002) *Health Action Zones: integrated case studies, preliminary findings*, Glasgow: University of Glasgow, Health Promotion Policy Unit.

Pawson, R. and Tilley, N. (1997) *Realistic evaluation*, London: Sage.

Section 1

Building capacity for collaboration in English Health Action Zones

Helen Sullivan, Marian Barnes and Elizabeth Matka

Introduction

Partnership and community involvement are central to the HAZ endeavour. From the outset partnership was considered a prerequisite to the development of local health strategies that would enable the resources of a wide variety of stakeholders, including central government, to be brought to bear on improving health and health services and reducing inequalities. Partnership was intended to include members of the community sector, either through community health councils, community and user organisations or through direct engagement with citizens. This reflected an agenda for community involvement that was about both recognising the contribution that citizens and users could make to problem identification and solution, and also requiring of citizens an acknowledgement of the responsibilities as well as the rights of citizenship (Barnes and Prior, 2000).

This commitment to partnership working and community involvement was reflected in central government's overarching principles for the operation of HAZs, two of which were:

- engaging communities – involving the public in planning services, and empowering service users and patients to take responsibility for their own health and decisions about care
- working in partnership – recognising that people receive services from a range of different agencies and that these services need to be coordinated to achieve the maximum benefit (DoH, 1997a).

One of the differences between the HAZ initiative and previous health partnerships was an expression of partnership that operated not only within localities but also between localities and the departments of government in pursuit of common goals. This was indicated in the invitation to bid for HAZ status in 1997: 'The centre will expect to work in partnership with the zone delivering support and "investment" against agreed milestones' (DoH, 1997b, 65).

This in turn reflected another New Labour impulse which was to modernise all aspects of public service. Here the HAZ was seen as an agent of change, creating the capacity to transform the local health system. By bringing professionals, communities and organisations together in the HAZ this would create the capacity for transformed service design and delivery within and beyond the health sphere.

The chapters contained in Section 1 illuminate the experience of local HAZs in developing and delivering through partnership and involving communities in their activities. They cover a wide range of HAZs and address the issues from a number of different perspectives. Holden and Craig (Chapter 1) critically reflect on the wide-ranging contribution made by community development to health in Hull/East Riding, while South and Green (Chapter 2) focus on the specific role played by community involvement specialists in influencing mainstream development in Bradford primary care groups (PCGs). Both of these papers are informed by participatory approaches to research. This theme is continued in the contributions of Sharpe et al. and Squires and Clark (Chapters 4 and 5), who explore the opportunities and challenges of research and evaluation that are undertaken by community members in contexts as diverse as Northumberland and Wolverhampton. A key theme emerging here relates to the skills and capacity generated through such initiatives. The account of the Salford Social Entrepreneurs Programme by Dabbs (Chapter 3) further develops this theme, and highlights the potential of individual interventions to benefit wider communities if learning generated in the programme can be sustained beyond its life. Learning is also a key aspect of the paper by Adams et al. (Chapter 6), which discusses the experiences of Wakefield HAZ in developing its partnership arrangements. These authors illustrate the power of the local context in helping or hindering collaboration. Finally, Halliday et al. (Chapter 7) draw on their experiences in Cornwall and the Isles of Scilly and Plymouth to consider the future, contemplating the possible contribution of the HAZ to the development of local strategic partnerships (LSPs).

The remainder of this introductory chapter provides context to these local case studies by drawing on the work of the national evaluation team responsible for considering 'building capacity for collaboration' across the HAZ community.

A national perspective

The 'theories of change' (Connell and Kubisch, 1998) approach to the evaluation being used by the national team emphasises the significance of the particular context within which strategies are being pursued, understanding context as both a source of opportunity and constraint. The team is posing the following evaluation questions, and carrying out work at strategic, meso and project level in each of five case study HAZs:

- What contribution does community involvement make to achieving HAZ objectives?
- What contribution do inter-agency partnerships make to achieving HAZ objectives?
- Can HAZs create the conditions in which community involvement meets the objectives of community participants, as well as those of statutory agencies?
- What is the contribution made by HAZs to the development of inter-agency partnerships as a mode of governance?

These questions acknowledge the need to understand both whether and how collaborative mechanisms can achieve the necessary changes, and whether the HAZ itself is an effective mechanism for building collaborative capacity. 'Theories of change' is helpful here as it requires HAZ partnerships to articulate the collaborative nature of the 'process–outcome' relationships within a 'whole systems' approach to health, including specifying the way in which community involvement activities will support the specified outcomes. It also requires HAZ partners to specify the type and level of collaborative capacity necessary to deliver HAZ objectives and to set about establishing these, to identify the key components necessary to build collaborative capacity and to identify how these will be resourced. Finally it forces a focus on the contribution of the HAZ to the achievement of wider community goals, thereby allowing for a number of perspectives to inform what is considered 'success'.

The material contained below is derived from a recent national evaluation report of the first year of the evaluation of building capacity for collaboration (Barnes et al., 2001). It draws on questionnaires, interviews and documentary material to start to explore context and strategies, to reflect on perceived capacity to pursue inter-agency partnerships and community involvement, and to identify learning and changes to date.

Context

There are two aspects to context that are of significance here. These are the influence of national context and the contribution of the 'locality effect'. All HAZs are operating within a national context which defines the parameters within which they work, offering opportunities but also imposing constraints. The national policy context towards the end of Labour's first term (end 2000/early 2001) was perceived by HAZ strategic stakeholders to be more favourable to the development of inter-agency collaboration and community involvement, in terms of the centrality of such mechanisms to the construction and implementation of policy, than had been the case in 1997. However, considerable constraints remained which mitigated such commitment. These were identified as: the pressure to achieve early wins, the number of policy initiatives launched by the government and the centralised performance management framework.

In addition to these contextual factors which will be familiar to those involved in previous attempts to build more effective collaboration across agencies and between statutory, voluntary and community sectors, the HAZ context offers three significant challenges to localities. The first pertains to the inherent complexity of the task facing HAZs. The HAZ initiative is far more ambitious than previous area-based health initiatives including a wider range of objectives and a much larger number of potential partners, at a time when partnership capacity is being tested to the limits by Labour's plethora of area-based initiatives (ABIs). Secondly, the HAZ was originally envisaged as a long-term initiative, which would have a major impact on the configuration and performance of the local health economy. This introduced a requirement for HAZs to contemplate how they would sustain such relationships, something that was confounded by the uncertainty introduced in relation to the future of HAZs after the 2001 election. Finally, while the idea of a new central–local partnership was broadly welcomed by local stakeholders, it did introduce an added tension to the relationship requiring localities to continue to enable bottom-up priorities and strategies to emerge, while also taking account of this vertical relationship.

National pressures, though powerful, are only part of the prevailing context. Their depth and resonance will be mediated in their interaction with local contextual factors, and it is this interaction which will give shape to the emergent local partnerships and processes for the HAZ. Therefore it is important that the particularity of the local context within which different HAZs are developing is examined and delineated. The key local factors emerging from the national evaluation's cross-HAZ analysis are:

- geographical tensions: managing inner/outer and urban/rural needs
- population change: managing the needs of stable and more mobile population cohorts
- population diversity
- the role of boundaries, in particular local authority boundaries and their relationship to HAZ boundaries

- political culture and relationships
- community identity and allegiance.

The particular configuration of these factors within localities helps explain why the HAZ initiative developed so differently across its 26 sites.

Strategy

The significance of partnership and community involvement to HAZ is reflected in the objectives of local HAZ strategies. There are four key objectives in relation to partnership working: achieving health improvements and reductions in health inequalities; the joint provision of improved services; systems of governance that are efficient and accountable; and more successful and embedded cross-agency and cross-sector working. In turn there are five objectives for community involvement: improving public accountability; improving health; improving services; accessing lay or experiential knowledge; and increasing public knowledge and support for the HAZ.

Evidence available to the national evaluation suggests that for these objectives to be achieved local strategies have to be active in five areas. At a *strategic level* action is necessary in order that the HAZ vision and its themes may be defined and developed. To inform the *governance* of the HAZ it is important to set in place decision-making processes and structures that will satisfy different accountability requirements, namely accountability upwards to the Department of Health and downwards to communities. To secure the successful implementation the key organisational structures and processes necessary to deliver, new activities must be delineated to support the HAZs' *operational capacity*. Staying with operational issues, any changes or reconfiguration of *practice* need to be determined, as do the core skills and abilities essential among workers in the HAZ. Finally action is essential among *communities and citizens*, specifically in relation to identifying and putting in place the cultural, material and personal resources for community members to take part in change processes.

The evaluation revealed four types of strategy within HAZs. While one strategy type predominated in any particular HAZ, elements of various strategies appeared alongside or at different times within HAZs.

The first type was the *consolidation strategy*. This focused upon taking stock of progress that had already been made and finding ways of building upon it. The rationale was that the problems and desired outcomes were well known and agreed, that previous activities had demonstrated some capacity to achieve outcomes, and that the purpose of the HAZ was to facilitate further progress by removing any existing obstacles and opening up new opportunities.

The work of Sandwell HAZ exemplified this strategy. Here the HAZ was viewed as a catalyst to draw programmes together and provide an opportunity to test out new ways of working. The approach used the HAZ to 'add value' to existing work wherever possible. The Health Partnership predated the HAZ and was considered likely to endure, whatever happened to the HAZ. The governance of the HAZ was through this mechanism, which was itself an arm of the borough's civic partnership.

The second strategy type was the *mainstreaming strategy*. This used the HAZ to secure mainstream change so that all organisations and sectors better understood their contribution to health and the infrastructure needed to support this. This strategy saw health as a cross-cutting issue which all sectors had a role in promoting. The HAZ was a powerful catalyst for change, but that change needed to be embedded in longer-term policy and delivery processes, such as Health Improvement Programmes (HImPs) and primary care groups/trusts.

The Bradford HAZ programme (Chapter 2) exemplified this kind of strategy. The emphasis on using the HAZ to support infrastructure change and development to take forward a more 'joined-up' agenda in relation to health was clear in the implementation plan. This manifested itself in a number of ways, such as the focus on collaboration at all levels from frontline to strategy: e.g. work with primary care groups and the use of HAZ resources to accelerate progress through the HImP, and the establishment of a community involvement team to work specifically at sub-locality level with primary care providers and communities to enhance their respective capacities.

The third strategy type was the *emergent strategy*. The emphasis here was to find the best way to deliver positive change in health improvement and health inequality in a complex and somewhat unfamiliar environment. The strategy derived from an acknowledgement that the HAZ entity was an artificial creation, and therefore the wholesale application of a single strategy was inappropriate and counterproductive. The particular needs and dynamics of the constituent parts of the HAZ required the application of different approaches. By testing out a range of different initiatives the HAZ could select which contributed to the development of a more robust strategy in the longer term.

The activities of Manchester, Salford and Trafford (MaST) HAZ illustrate the operation of this strategy in practice. Initial attempts to work in a client-based HAZ-wide manner proved difficult, in part because of the need to establish HAZ-wide systems and processes to facilitate working across this area. The HAZ subsequently set about working in a more targeted manner, within development sites in local authority areas and through trailblazing policy or service-specific initiatives. The governance arrangements for partnership in the HAZ followed a similar pattern, with initial attempts to develop an all-embracing framework replaced by a more streamlined partnership board with considerable devolution to the operational levels.

The final strategy type we identified was the *innovation strategy*. This focused on a particular aspect of the HAZ agenda – innovation – to challenge conventional approaches. The strategy's rationale was that in order to genuinely transform prevailing policy and practice, a widespread surge of innovation was necessary to establish momentum for change but also to test out and assess a variety of new approaches.

Lambeth, Southwark and Lewisham (LSL) HAZ exemplified an attempt to develop and apply a strategy initially oriented toward innovation. Their implementation plan Children First emphasised the need to focus on preventative work with children and families in order to secure the necessary changes in service provision, access and use to facilitate improved life chances. The governance arrangements for the HAZ tried to reflect this emphasis on innovation by specifying a key role for cross-organisational programme groups (existing below the partnership board and alongside the executive group) to commission projects in line with the principles of Children First. The original strategy resulted in the commissioning of a large number of projects. The HAZ was seen as a body separate from existing agencies with the role of influencing the mainstream from outside, rather than working through mainstream agencies.

In each case the HAZ strategy that initially emerged was informed by the prevailing local context. The extent to which the HAZ strategies changed over time was based upon the experience of implementation and importantly the changing national agenda. Within the two coterminous HAZs with which we have been working, Bradford and Sandwell, the overall strategy remained largely consistent during the life of the HAZ, but the two multi-authority HAZs (MaST and LSL) made significant changes to their strategic direction during the life of the HAZ.

Capacity

Whether the HAZs had sufficient capacity to achieve their objectives in relation to partnership and community involvement was a core question for the national evaluation. We found that the partnership capacity of HAZs was affected by a number of factors. The first pertained to its legitimacy. The more it was considered a credible agent 'owned' by the key stakeholders the greater its legitimacy. A consistently important issue was the nature of the power relationships within the HAZ. Status between partners to the HAZ was not perceived to be equal, something that voluntary sector partners perceived particularly keenly. This was linked to the third factor, the capacity of the individual partners to contribute to the HAZ. While most partners were aware of the necessary skills and capacities needed to work in partnership, some found it difficult to release that capacity because of other pressures on their organisations. In some cases HAZ resourcing was directed towards helping support voluntary and community bodies to participate in strategic forums. However, for other sectors, e.g. the private sector, partnership working in relation to HAZ was frequently too time-consuming.

The degree to which partners understood the HAZ as a separate 'stand-alone' entity also influenced partnership capacity. In some cases the concept of the HAZ had become linked specifically to a core 'HAZ team'. Here partners sometimes experienced irritation with what they perceived to be interference by the HAZ in their core activities. Finally partnership capacity was also affected by the development of wider collaborative relationships between partners. Where the HAZ had provided entry for partners to new arenas and opportunities, most often in relation to regeneration, its capacity was increased and perceptions of its utility also rose.

The perception of capacity in relation to community involvement highlighted a number of factors. There was evidence of variation in the extent to which partners shared a collective view of the purpose or purposes of community involvement. For example, for some there were clear differences between objectives related to community involvement and community development, while for others the two were used interchangeably. The extent to which the development of HAZ plans had been informed by community involvement was also contested. For some this was not perceived to be the most significant feature of community involvement, while for others engagement at the strategic-planning stage was critical to involving communities as key partners. We found that most of the effort in terms of building capacity for community involvement was focused at project or sub-local level – there was limited evidence of increasing capacity for community involvement at strategic level. However, this was accompanied by some indications that this might not be a priority for voluntary and community partners. Community capacity building was considered to be under-resourced as an activity in HAZs, thus preventing the empowerment of communities across a range of groups/areas. Finally some ways of working within HAZs were considered to exclude those who did not know the 'rules of the game'– though there was also evidence that HAZs were acknowledging and seeking to address this.

Change

Change was evident in a number of areas in relation to partnership working and community involvement in the HAZ. Changes identified related to the nature of what could be done under the HAZ that could not be done elsewhere. So the HAZ was cited as funding 'risky' issues or targeting groups who would not be prioritised within mainstream service delivery agencies. Here it could act as a learning laboratory, testing new ways of doing things with a view to main-streaming them if they were successful. Changes in the way in which people work together, informally as well as through more formal processes, were fre-quently reported as resulting from the application of HAZ strategies. Getting health on the agenda of other regeneration programmes and partnerships was also a welcome change, as was the degree to which HAZ activity was shaping the emergent LSPs. Finally, there was some evidence of the HAZ's shaping and influencing the development of mainstream services and policy initiatives. One clear example of this is the work of Bradford HAZ in developing the PCG/T role in community involvement.

A key dilemma for HAZs, however, pertained to attribution. It was frequently not possible to attribute particular changes to the HAZ alone, particularly in a context in which HAZs were seeking to work with other initiatives and in which the boundary of 'HAZ' was fluid and fuzzy.

Conclusion

At the time of writing the evaluation of HAZs is ongoing, so it is inappropriate to offer any firm conclusions. However, it is possible to identify some emerging issues associated with building capacity for collaboration in HAZs.

It is clear that collaborative capacity in all its forms is key to successful part-nership development and community involvement. However, both activities take considerable time, and those HAZs that have experienced most difficulty are those that have least collective collaborative memory to draw upon. Partnership working with particular sectors requires tailored effort: for example, private sector organisations have to be engaged in something tangible, and com-munities need to be involved at the point at which collaboration makes most sense to them. Similarly, community involvement is not a generic activity but one that needs to be sensitive to the particular community that is being engaged.

Power relationships and power imbalances are critically important in attempts to build partnerships and involve communities in collaborative effort. In relation to partnership the biggest gaps are between the statutory and non-statutory sec-tors, with communities having the least leverage. The resource power of key bod-ies such as health providers and local authorities is central to this imbalance, as is the relative commonality of interest between health and social services based upon past experience of working together. In relation to community involve-ment there is a clear message that without adequate resourcing in terms of capac-ity building and support, communities cannot be full partners, and that particular attention needs to be paid to those communities that are unlikely to form organised groups and are constantly marginalised.

At a local level, partnership is now generally accepted as an important way of working to achieve key outcomes. However, there remain difficulties associated with developing and sustaining partnerships over time. Specific tensions emerged in partnerships where mechanisms for decision making and supervision were perceived to be too cumbersome by partners used to more efficient mechanisms, and too exclusive by those partners used to extensive systems for accountability. These performance/conformance tensions are likely to remain key issues in a governance environment that prioritises efficiency and involvement equally.

However, an overriding message from HAZs to date is that it is not possible to understand local partnerships divorced from their national context, nor expect them to deliver if national policy is not moving in the same direction. While the national agenda is more conducive to partnership working and community involvement, the dynamics of the national policy context are such that it is not possible for localities to be confident that national government will be able to follow through the implications of its agenda for collaborative action at the local level.

References

Barnes, M. and Prior, D. (2000) *Private lives as public policy*, Birmingham: Venture Press.

Barnes, M., Sullivan, H. and Matka, E. (2001) *Building capacity for collaboration: the national evaluation of Health Action Zones, context, strategy and capacity: initial findings from the strategic level analysis, HAZ strategic overview report*, Birmingham: University of Birmingham.

Connell, J. P. and Kubisch, A. C. (1998) 'Applying a theory of change approach to the evaluation of comprehensive community initiatives: progress, prospects, and problems', in Fulbright-Anderson, K., Kubisch, A. C. and Connell, J. P. (eds) *New approaches to evaluating community initiatives*, vol. 2, *Theory, measurement, and analysis*, Washington, DC: The Aspen Institute, 15–44.

DoH (1997a) *£30 million for new partnerships to target health inequalities*, Press Release no. 312, October, Department of Health.

DoH (1997b) *Health Action Zones: invitation to bid*, EL(97)65, 30 October, Leeds: Department of Health.

CHAPTER 1

Engaging communities in the Hull/East Riding Health Action Zone: the role of community development in addressing health inequalities

Sue Holden and Gary Craig

The Hull and East Riding Health Action Zone (HERHAZ) is a second-wave HAZ, starting in 1999, within a local context illustrating well the links between poverty, inequality and ill health, and the growing divide between more healthy and less healthy areas (DoH, 2001a,b; Shaw et al., 2001). It incorporates starkly deprived areas of urban deprivation (Hull is, depending on the measure used – low income, unemployment, ill health – around the thirteenth most-deprived authority in England and Wales) alongside a rural area that has pockets of deprivation but also has serious problems of access to services and facilities (DETR, 2000). The contrast between Kingston upon Hull and the East Riding of Yorkshire has provided an additional challenge, as the expectations of the HAZ are that it will offer innovative and locally effective projects. The wide range of projects created and supported by the HAZ has met that challenge. These vary from the introduction of a Healthy Living Centre concept to Hull Prison, to the Rural Stress Initiative supporting farmers and their families through recent agricultural crises. It was agreed in early meetings of the local HAZ evaluation group that the community development workstream should be one major focus of the university-based evaluation work, alongside work on tobacco cessation, intermediate care and sexual health promotion.

Evaluation and community development

There is a growing literature on the theoretical and value base of community development, and of techniques for evaluating its complexities, reflected in an initial paper (Craig, 2000a) presented to the HERHAZ Evaluation Steering Group. Hughes and Traynor (2000) also identify some key issues. The first is timescale: they argue that 'community development professionals believe that the process of regeneration needs many years' work, and that policy-makers and policy evaluators under-represent this; in their turn, the latter may wonder whether such an assertion is in part due to their reluctance to examine rigorously the effectiveness of community interventions', a criticism which might apply to the instigators of the HAZ programme. A second key issue is causality or 'how you can clearly attribute change or growth to the social intervention. Such evaluative techniques as have been developed in this field cannot absolutely exclude other causality' (ibid.). Rossi and Freeman (1989) also offer a typology of five 'confounding factors' which limit attribution of change in community development evaluation.

A third complication for the evaluator – and of concern to all interested parties – is the difficulty of collecting credible data. It is usually the case that each will have a different concept of what constitutes success, and of what appropriate indicators might be. The fourth difficulty in community development evaluation is linked to each of the first three, namely the emphasis that is necessarily placed on process. An initiative may appear to reach the intended outcome, but the work may have been done in such a way that the community does not own it, and therefore it does not achieve sustainability. This is not a successful outcome in community development terms.

These complexities are well understood by the community health development (CHD) workers now working for HERHAZ. They are aware that some of their work has been slowly developing even in fertile soil (community development work is not new to the area). They are aware also of the need for long-term investment, and that successful outcomes they are now reaching often have roots in past work which has privileged a commitment to working in an empowering way with communities.

Weiss (1995) and Connell and Kubisch (1996) have expanded the knowledge and application of the 'theories of change' approach to the evaluation of social programmes. Weiss argues that evaluation should be theory-based because: (1) it focuses the evaluation on key aspects of the programme; (2) it enables the results from evaluation to be fed into wider knowledge of such programmes; (3) it requires operational staff to be explicit about their assumptions; and (4) it is therefore likely to be more influential in addressing policy and opinion. Our experience has also been that it has enabled positive links to be made between process and outcomes, as well as between theory and practice. We have also learnt that where theory has not been used to structure discussion about objectives, outcomes and indicators, there are inconsistent and unrealistic expectations of evaluation.

The HAZ National Evaluation Team also uses realistic evaluation theory (Pawson and Tilley, 1997) to add to the theories of change in their approach. In the local evaluation of the HERHAZ community development programme, evaluation theory derived from realistic evaluation, theories of change, and components from the 'ABCD model' (Barr et al., 1996a,b) of evaluation for community development have been used as a framework when possible, and valued by the local evaluators. Their approach has generally been within the action–research paradigm, with the evaluation team additionally engaging in policy discussions regarding the development of community development work locally where that seemed appropriate.

The HERHAZ Evaluation Steering Group committed itself to a form of participatory evaluation of community development work from the outset, accepting that this expressed the importance of the process of community development work itself. One of the most influential sets of guidelines for the evaluation of community development is to be found in the ABCD handbook, which states:

> In keeping with the principles, values, and definitions of community development, evaluation in this area needs to be developed through a participatory process. This means that all stakeholders should have a say in what should be measured and how that measurement should be undertaken and presented. In addition stakeholders should be encouraged to use their own knowledge and data already collected to provide the data required.
>
> Barr and Hashagen, 2000

Our research with local community development workers has therefore striven to mirror the consultative style of the community development workers with their communities.

Barr et al. also identify measures and building blocks which express the differing components of community development (see also Craig, 2000b). These can be used to provide a framework for the collection of information relevant to seeking indicators for change taking place in a community. This framework has been developed by Barr and Hashagen in the ABCD guidelines on evaluation and adopted in the strategic framework produced by the Standing Conference on Community Development (SCCD, 2001). This is of course by no means the first major attempt at community development work in a health context, but it may be the first time it has been subjected to rigorous independent evaluation (*CDJ*, 1993; Jones, 1999).

Community development in HERHAZ

Labonte (1997) discusses the need for health professionals to form genuine alliances with the communities they serve. His argument relates to the place of the community development approach in public health work:

community health thinking today represents an invitation we have made to ourselves to re-humanise, re-socialise and politicise our work. There is now an acknowledgement that the most important determinants of health, and disease, do not lie in medical or even behavioural health interventions, but in the quality of sharing and caring in our communities, and in how our social systems structure either fairness and equality, or unfairness and inequality. (See also Hashagen, 1998)

The initial HERHAZ implementation plan identified community development as one of its key 'workstream' areas, and listed desired outcomes:

- increased local input into local strategies which can impact on health
- increased awareness of the holistic concept of health
- actions taken to address social determinants of health
- a community development approach adopted by organisations
- sustainability – an aim shared throughout all HAZ projects.

The initial discussion paper by Craig (2000a) was agreed to by the HERHAZ Evaluation Steering Group as establishing a framework for both developing and evaluating community development work. The paper offered an inclusive definition of community development, and a three-tiered framework for thinking about the roles that community development might play within the context of a programme driven by emphases on addressing health inequalities through a participatory approach. The three-tiered approach was as follows:

i provision of resources for direct community development work (essentially this became focused on the employment of five community health development workers) – the goal of *local community empowerment* (Craig and Mayo, 1995)
ii indirect support for existing community development activity – the goal of *building infrastructural activity and professional development*
iii ensuring that the community development philosophy came to be reflected within the work of other agencies, particularly those concerned with primary health interventions – the goal of *policy and service delivery influence.*

Progress in these areas is discussed below, focusing in particular on the direct community health development work.

Provision of direct resources

The HAZ established an early funding stream to employ community development workers focusing on health issues within defined geographical areas where differing local health issues might emerge. Five workers are now in post. There are four primary care trust (PCT) areas locally, two in the very substantially deprived city of Hull and two in East Yorkshire, a very large semi-rural unitary authority with significant pockets of deprivation. The workers are based in PCT offices and cover PCT areas except in Yorkshire Wolds and Coast, (a huge area geographically), where there are two workers. One of these is based in the PCT office and the other in Bridlington in a new Community Resource Centre. One PCT area, West Hull, has had three different people in the post during the eighteen-month period for which it has existed, and progress here has therefore been particularly difficult to evaluate.

The job description for the CHD workers bravely embraced all basic elements in Craig's definition of community development, rather than the more limited aspects of developing participation. The management and support structure for this group of workers is unusual and merits explanation. The workers are funded by the HAZ until March 2002, but they are managed within the PCT. At the same time, because it was feared that they might have little common ground in the PCT with other health service workers, it was felt important that they obtained professional development support from community development experts, including guidance on philosophy, approaches, and skills development, as well as opportunities for them to share experiences with each other. Their brief also encompassed ensuring the development of the HAZ Community Development Programme, and its coordination with other agencies. The Community Development Foundation (CDF) was appointed to undertake these tasks in liaison with the community development evaluation team.

Semi-structured interviews were conducted with the CHD workers during their first six months in post. These were, firstly, to review basic demographic and other quantitative data for their area, and to brief them on information from the *Index of multiple deprivation* (DETR, 2000). This also enabled the team to assess any other information the workers had about their areas, generally little at that stage. The combination of information thus assembled did, however, give the workers a detailed breakdown of key needs of their areas, and this, together with some of their developing knowledge of local facilities, has proved useful. This again pointed to the considerable contrast, in terms of both demography and deprivation, between Kingston upon Hull and East Yorkshire, particularly in the Yorkshire Wolds and Coast area.

A second round of interviews with CHD workers looked at their attitudes, approaches and values, and examined their understanding of the various parts of community development work, broadly working to the definition accepted by the HERHAZ Evaluation Steering Group:

Community development is a way of working with people which starts with the needs and aspirations of groups of disadvantaged people in poor and deprived communities (whether socially or geographically defined). It struggles to articulate and organise politically (in the broadest sense) around these needs and aspirations, placing them at the front rather than at the end of political and policy debate. It strives to give ordinary people a voice for expressing and acting on their needs and desires and, through a process of participating in this approach to social change, offers people (again often the most powerless and deprived) support for their empowerment.

Craig, 2000a

In relation to systematic evaluation of outcomes, the evaluation team looked particularly at the work of Barr et al. (1996a,b). In addition, they began to collect information about the CHD work at the level of individuals, groups and projects. Consultative meetings were undertaken with the CHD workers as a group, first to discuss with them intended outcomes, and to consider possible indicators for those outcomes. CHD workers have also advised extensively on the questionnaire used for semi-structured interviews held with PCT chief executives and other health service managers to establish the latter's knowledge of and commitment to community development work. Although meetings with CHD workers have had explicit agendas to work to, in relation to evaluation of their own work, they also were important in developing a sense of solidarity and shared interests across the five very different areas in which work was being undertaken. Some early observations can be made.

- The underlying theme uniting the work of this group is that the workers clearly endorse 'the importance of seeing community development as a bottom-up process, focusing on the most disempowered members of the community'. The CHD workers have all discussed the importance of listening to people in community development work, and enabling people to be heard in policy and planning arenas of the NHS.

- The CHD workers are becoming organisationally absorbed into the PCT structure. Two of the four posts have been made permanent on becoming vacant. The second very nearly became a (somewhat diluted) 'participation worker', but there are special circumstances for that area. The three remaining posts appear to have full support from their PCT chief executives, although it remains to be seen if this is will still be the case when the HAZ funding ceases. This puts community development potentially at the heart of new primary health developments, and, if continuing organisation support for this work comes about, may represent a great achievement for the HAZ in terms of establishing the importance of local communities as key actors in health policy, service and practice development.

- The CHD workers are committed to the wider agenda and understandings of inequalities in health (Marmot and Wilkinson, 1999), and to using the same criteria and approaches as other community development workers based outside the health service. They are as likely to be involved in supporting a group of mothers to create a holiday period playground in a cul-de-sac on housing estates as they are to be supporting healthy lifestyle activity such as 'extend' (exercise for older people). Given this broader understanding of community health, our observation is that, given an innovative managerial approach, the setting in which the worker is based and the geography of the area have more influence over the choice of project worked with than the formal title of the worker. However, the title and organisational location of the workers obviously affect the policy and service implications of the outcomes of their work.

- The workers all express clear community development values, and share the definitions of community development accepted by the HAZ, seeing community development as a philosophical approach as well as a methodology with a set of identifiable skills.

- They do not all provide the same kind of service or work in the same detailed way. One works in a large rural area with no large centres of population and few pockets of deprivation. The most pressing need to be met for this area is that of improving access to services. This worker has focused on participation in her work, and building local sustainable community organisations. By contrast, another works in the most deprived area of Kingston upon Hull, covering the tenth most-deprived ward for families in England. She focuses most on confidence and capacity building with individuals and groups.

- All the workers believe it is an important part of their job to encourage organisations they work with to adopt the community development approach in the planning and delivery of health services. One PCT manager is concerned to ensure that community development as a 'philosophical approach' is practised throughout his PCT. However, there are different levels of understanding of the term 'community development' held by different organisations or individuals to whom they are accountable, or from whom they receive advice and support.

- The workers are all involved in a variety of community development projects in their areas, some more so than others. This includes for each of them projects that attract funding to their areas, such as Healthy Living Centre bids, and Sure Start developments. They are all involved in community activist training, and have developed partnerships with local regeneration or community schemes. They work with inequalities of all sorts, including promoting projects that enable communities to get to know and accept asylum seekers.

One example is the cookery classes held by local women in a West Hull community centre, introducing their new neighbours to English food.

- There are many encouraging examples of the HAZ community development workstream initiating and supporting changes which appear to result in a reduction of inequalities in health, and to be sustainable, although it is too early to characterise these as firm (and possibly quantifiable) outcomes. Large numbers of young men have quit smoking for more than a month in Hull Prison, following the introduction by the East Hull CHD worker of the Laryngectomy Society to their health information sessions. Health information days have been well attended throughout the HAZ, and at the internet café established in Bridlington for young people. This has a good chance of attracting European funding for next year. Several of the projects undertaken, including the internet café, have followed participatory appraisals. The Bridlington Sure Start Management Group is organised by parents who have developed skills and confidence to manage a task that local politicians expected and were expected to do. This took some of the politicians by surprise, but this transition was well handled by the local East Riding Council partnerships manager. Her involvement with the health authority 'Support for Community Development' meetings has also enabled her to share the significance of this piece of work on a wider basis. Elsewhere in the East Riding, the Riley Theatre presented *Living with a teenager*, which was very well received in local and other venues by audiences of adults and teenagers. This performance was the result of a partnership between the CHD workers, the Education Action Zone, and the police, and successfully portrayed in a non-threatening way some of the very perplexing problems that face young people and their parents today. All the CHD workers have been involved in healthy eating (Fit, Funky Food) and in exercise projects. They are also involved in forums and patient/public participation groups.

Indirect support for existing community development activity

This is the goal originally described to HERHAZ as 'building infrastructural capacity' but, for the CHD workers, it is also particularly concerned with professional development and support. One of the best examples of this work in action in the HAZ is the Community Chest, prefiguring a scheme being introduced under the government's neighbourhood renewal scheme. The HAZ Community Chest gives grants to local organisations of up to £500 (totalling £25,000 in a year), many of them supporting community development activities. Decisions are made by CHD workers together with the HAZ development manager.

The HEROS website (www.heros.org.uk/) is another HAZ-funded scheme, forming the core of its Public Information Programme. The website contains information about the Hull and East Riding area, including the Community Development Directory, a list of community development schemes in the area compiled by the HERHAZ community development evaluation team for the community development workstream. This Directory has been used, for example, to disseminate information about a conference on energy conservation held in the East Riding, and for networking.

One of the most important examples of indirect support for existing community development is the support and professional development work offered by the Community Development Foundation to the CHD workers. The CDF also supports the HAZ Community Development Programme more generally, including taking part in organising a major subregional conference on community development held in Hull which aimed to invest local activity with a new sense of purpose and partnership. A proposal has been put to the conference organisers that one medium-term outcome should be a subregional community development forum covering the whole of Humberside, tasked to support the development and promotion of local community development work at all levels, through support for training, information, networking, conferences, seminars and workshops. This would offer the opportunity for CHD workers to build stronger links with other local CD workers.

Ensuring the community development philosophy is reflected within the work of other, particularly health-related, agencies

The working definition of community development adopted by HERHAZ (Craig, 2000a) legitimates work which focuses on bringing about organisational change. It requires community development to include capacity building, involvement of individuals and groups in defining their own needs, leading to active participation and contributing to service and policy development. It recognises the requirement for organisations to evolve, by opening up structures and systems to address community needs as defined and expressed by the community, defined both by geography and interest. It identifies the process of empowerment as critical – 'the creation of sustainable structures, processes and mechanisms, over which communities have an increased degree of control, and which themselves have a measurable impact on public and social policy affecting those communities'. Above all, the definition used includes as a key principle the importance of seeing community development as a 'bottom-up' process, focusing on the most disempowered members of the community.

To evaluate this process of policy and service change, each worker was asked how they saw their role in bringing about organisational change. All felt that it was part of their work to bring the PCTs to adopt the ethos of community development. They felt they had opportunities to influence in the feedback sessions they had, and that their management support arrangements gave them access to significant decision-making groups. Some could give concrete examples of changes they had brought about. One CHD worker had gained a proper acknowledgement for the costs incurred by users and carers who attended meetings to help with the design of forms. The workers have now started to bring out a three-monthly well-produced newspaper to inform health service workers and other agencies about all the community development activities that are taking place in their area.

Again, it is too early to talk about sustainable outcomes in terms of organisational change. Certainly, within a series of meetings involving wide-ranging organisational interests and convened by the health authority, there has been growing understanding of the full meaning of the term 'community development' and the implications for health services managers of absorbing the community development philosophy into their structures, often for the first time. This perception will be tested in interviews with key actors towards the end of the evaluation to see how this understanding is reflected in changing organisational practices and policy. As noted above, PCT managers are coming to endorse the value of long-term community development work. The CDF is playing a role in offering community development management training to managers of CHD workers. The evaluation will continue to examine these issues to provide a rounded view of the impact of community development work both directly and indirectly in addressing health inequalities.

Throughout the HERHAZ Community Development Programme there are encouraging signs of progress towards the achievement of the HAZ aims and intended outcomes. The evaluation will continue to monitor progress into the middle of 2002. This still constitutes a very short timescale within which to establish the sustainability of identified changes, by the time the evaluative work comes to an end with the write-up of findings (by December 2002). It may at least provide some preliminary pointers to future work in these important and developing areas of community health development work.

References

Barr, A. and Hashagen, S. (2000) *ABCD handbook*, London: Community Development Foundation

Barr, A., Hashagen, S. and Purcell, R. (1996a) *Measuring community development in Northern Ireland: a handbook for practitioners*, Glasgow: Scottish Community Development Centre.

Barr, A., Hashagen, S. and Purcell, R. (1996b) *Monitoring and evaluation of community development in Northern Ireland,* Glasgow: Scottish Development Centre.

CDJ (1993) *Community Development Journal,* 28/3 [special issue on control of health care].

Connell, J. and Kubisch A. (eds) (1996) *Evaluating comprehensive community initiatives,* Washington, DC: Aspen Institute.

Craig, G. (2000a) *Supporting, initiating and evaluating community development in the Hull/East Riding Health Action Zone,* Hull: University of Hull, Mimeo. [copies available from G.Craig@hull.ac.uk].

Craig, G. (2000b) *What works in community development with children?,* Ilford: Barnardo's.

Craig, G. and Mayo, M. (1995) *Community empowerment: a reader in participation and development,* London: Zed Books.

DETR (2000) *Index of multiple deprivation,* London: The Stationery Office/Department of the Environment, Transport and the Regions.

DoH (2001a) *From vision to reality,* London: The Stationery Office/Department of Health.

DoH (2001b*) Tackling health inequalities,* London: The Stationery Office/Department of Health.

Hashagen, S. (1998) *Community development and health,* Edinburgh: HEBS/University of Edinburgh.

Hughes, M. and Traynor, T. (2000) 'Reconciling process and outcome in evaluating community initiatives', *Evaluation,* 6/1, 37–49.

Jones, J. (1999) *Private troubles and public issues: a community development approach to health,* Edinburgh: Community Learning Scotland.

Labonte, R. (1997) 'Community and public health: an international perspective', *Health Visitor,* 70, 64–7.

Marmot, M. and Wilkinson, R. G. (eds) (1999) *Social determinants of health,* Oxford: Oxford University Press.

Pawson, R. and Tilley, N. (1997) *Realistic evaluation,* London: Sage.

Rossi, P. H. and Freeman, H. E. (1989) *Evaluation: a systematic approach,* Newbury Park, CA: Sage.

SCCD (2001) *Strategic framework for community development,* Sheffield: Standing Conference on Community Development.

Shaw, M., Dorling, D. and Smith, G. D. (2001) *Mind the gap: inequalities continue to widen under New Labour,* Bristol: University of Bristol [http://www.social-medicine.com/townrep.html].

Weiss, C. H. (1995) 'Nothing as practical as good theory: exploring theory based evaluation of comprehensive community initiatives for children and families', in Connell, J. P., Kubisch, A. C., Schorr, L. B. and Weiss, C. H. (eds) *New approaches to evaluating community initiatives: concepts, method and context,* Washington, DC: Aspen Institute.

CHAPTER 2

Building community involvement in primary care trusts: an evaluation of a Health Action Zone Community Involvement Team in Bradford

Jane South and Eleanor Green

Bradford is a metropolitan district covering both urban and rural areas and encompassing diverse communities, including a large minority ethnic population. Deprivation exists in many areas of the city and there is significant poor health in the district. A commitment to tackle health inequalities, a history of inter-agency partnership working and support for community development approaches made Bradford in some ways a 'natural' for HAZ status. The question was how to use the HAZ to build on existing community development work and achieve greater community involvement in health planning and decision making. One of the key approaches taken was to establish a specialist team to work with the new primary care groups (PCGs) to help them to engage with their local communities. This chapter examines why this approach was adopted, what has happened since in the PCGs, what lessons have been learnt and how the work will be taken forward. The term 'community involvement' as used in this chapter refers to the participation of local geographic communities, communities of interest, service users and carers, and the general public.

Context and rationale

Bradford was one of the first-wave Health Action Zones and, like other areas, HAZ status created an opportunity to further existing work in community involvement and strengthen partnership working. A period of strategic development across different sectors to support greater public and user participation in planning and service development, much of it driven by national policy, was already creating a mandate for change in the district. The decision to develop and fund a specialist district team to promote community involvement in health was informed by the need to convert those strategic intentions into actions. Research commissioned by the HAZ Partnership Board had shown that there was a significant amount of community and voluntary activity across the district, but a more coordinated approach to involvement and improved communication between agencies and communities was required (Wilson, 1999).

In this context what was needed was to join up existing activity and to develop the capacity of statutory organisations to listen and respond to local communities, communities of interest and service users. A decision was made to establish a district Community Involvement Team, which would be funded through the HAZ. The overall aims of the team were:

1 to strengthen the capacity of PCGs to involve communities in health and health care planning, decision making and delivery
2 to strengthen the capacity of communities to participate in health and health care planning, decision making and delivery.

The local context meant that the HAZ Community Involvement Team would mainly work with community development workers and other allies, rather than working directly with communities. The principal focus of the work was on building capacity in the new PCGs. It was envisaged that the team would be key actors in creating and maintaining links between the PCGs and the community and voluntary sectors. At the time of the establishment of the team, Bradford had four PCGs, which later all became primary care trusts (PCTs). The then PCGs were new health organisations with specific responsibilities for meeting the needs of local populations that they served. It was recognised that these organisations would eventually have considerable power and resources within the health family as they took over responsibility for the commissioning and delivery of care. Their establishment, therefore, presented a unique opportunity to build community involvement into the mainstream business and cultural fabric of key health organisations as they developed.

The team starts

The HAZ Community Involvement Team was established in 1999, funded for two years from the HAZ. Recruitment of the team followed the appointment of the team manager in September 1999, and the last member came into post in February 2000. The team consisted of a manager and four team members who were each linked to one of Bradford's PCGs. Team members had a variety of prior experience, including community development work, health promotion, and work concerning disability and other equal opportunities issues. Two were from minority ethnic communities. In order to promote coordination and partnership working the team has been managed within the local authority's Neighbourhood Support Service, which aims to provide a bridge between the council and local communities through a network of neighbourhood forums.

The innovative nature of the team's work and the predicted challenges involved in promoting a huge cultural change in health care organisations meant that it was important to know what worked, what difficulties arose and what lessons could be learnt. A collaborative evaluation, with Bradford University, Bradford Health Authority and the team, was set up to run concurrently with the team's initial funding period. An action evaluation approach (Fawcett, 2000) was adopted, which has allowed team members and other stakeholders to reflect on practice, and use the findings to inform the development of the work. Multiple methods are being used in order to capture the views of different stakeholders, including community perspectives. The findings presented here are drawn from the first stage of data collection. The main sources of data were: reports documenting activities, completed bimonthly by team members; unstructured interviews with team members; and semi-structured interviews with sixteen individuals working in the four PCTs, either as managers or as professional executive committee (PEC) members. A thematic analysis of all interview data was carried out.

Ways of working

The work of the Bradford HAZ Community Involvement Team has been primarily about capacity building and joining up existing community activity. Although the initial focus was on organisational development in the four PCTs, the team has also worked in localities and district-wide to build links between statutory organisations and community/voluntary groups. It has not done this alone but in collaboration with other organisations and teams supporting community development infrastructure.

Monitoring reports indicate the range and diversity of activities undertaken by team members, and the number of organisations and groups that they have had contact with. Box 2.1 gives some examples of activities to illustrate the range of work. In summary, their work takes place at a strategic level, working with others to build infrastructure for involvement, through to supporting local groups and forums.

Box 2.1 Examples of activities

Activities undertaken by members of the Bradford HAZ Community Involvement Team:

- developing a PCT equality and diversity strategy

- organising a networking day to bring together all members of the local HAZ family, including funded projects, in one PCT area and hold training on communication

- working with a Healthy Living Centre bid to facilitate links between the 31 agencies and communities within the partnership, and securing funding to enable the bid to progress. A senior manager from the PCT now sits on the development team

- carrying out an audit of patient and public involvement in general practices and then working with individual practices to develop activities

- helping set up and maintain a men's health group working with Asian young men.

The team's role in the primary care trusts

It was intended that the team would work with others to build organisational capacity so that the four PCTs could begin to engage with their local communities. In other words, the team was to have an enabling role as opposed to 'doing it' for the PCTs. The specific mix of activities undertaken has varied between individual team members but the evaluation found that key aspects of the team's role are broadly similar. The key aspects are: an educative role, building links between the PCTs and local groups, and capacity building in the organisation.

The team's educative role

Team members are perceived as having a crucial role in raising awareness within the PCTs and also with primary health care staff. One GP described the team member as a bit of a champion 'flying the flag' for community involvement. A low level of knowledge about community involvement and some degree of apprehension concerning what it meant for PCTs and primary care was reported in the early days. Team members have worked to increase understanding of community involvement, highlight its importance and offer practical suggestions as to how it can be integrated into practice.

Building links

Networking and building links with communities have been regarded by those in the PCTs as perhaps the most significant and valued aspect of the team's role. The evaluation has shown that team members have initiated contact and responded to requests from a large number of different organisations, groups and individuals. Links have been built between communities and the PCTs in a variety of ways. On one level, team members have acted as an access point for community groups, while on another level, team members have had a role in preparation and support for participatory processes, either within the PCT or in other partnerships.

An important part of the team's work has been about supporting the involvement of groups and individuals who are traditionally under-represented, and this has included work to support greater participation of black and minority ethnic communities. This has particular significance for City PCT, where over half the population are from ethnic minorities. The team member there has on many occasions acted as an essential bridge between the PCT and those communities. In all the PCTs it has been recognised that time and effort are required in order to build relationships with all communities, and that team members have made an essential contribution to this.

Capacity building

The importance of the team member's role in building infrastructure for involvement within the organisation has also been recognised. Activities have included developing patient and public involvement strategies, identifying resources, developing participatory structures, and ensuring that there are robust and supportive commissioning processes for funding community projects.

Overall the evaluation found that the team's role is valued in the PCTs. Many of those interviewed considered that the team's contribution has in fact been essential. Early work to build credibility for the team and the community involvement agenda in the PCTs appears to have paid off. The potential for a team member to be seen as the person who 'does' community involvement has not been realised: instead there is a clear understanding in PCTs of the enabling nature of the role. Team members were often described as a 'resource' and their expertise is recognised, particularly their skills in accessing local networks and groups.

Moving forward

A specialist resource having been provided, a question for the evaluation was whether progress had been made in getting greater community involvement in planning, decision making and delivery of health and health care. The findings indicate that all four PCTs in Bradford have begun to grapple with the realities of implementing community involvement. This is in the context of considerable organisational change, including moving from PCG to PCT status. In addition, during this period national policy has promoted greater patient and public involvement in the health service (NHS Executive, 1999; DoH, 2001). Inevitably the work of the team has been integrated with the PCTs' response to this agenda.

There is evidence of a great deal of commitment to the principle of community involvement in the four PCTs, and this was reported both by those with a role in community involvement and also those with responsibilities for other areas of work. Maintaining it on the agenda appears to be the result of a number of different players' efforts, and can undoubtedly be seen as an achievement in the context of competing priorities and huge workloads.

The necessity of cultural change is key to the whole business of integrating community involvement into mainstream work. There has been some evidence that the PCTs, as new organisations, are beginning to develop cultures that are supportive of community involvement. Issues of shared responsibility and making community involvement integral to practice are considered important. Work has been taking place on clinical governance and developing community involvement targets for practices. Many of those interviewed, however, highlighted the continuing need to raise awareness of community involvement in general practice, and help primary health care staff tune into new ways of working with patients and the public.

Although community involvement is a shared aspiration within the four PCTs, there is a general perception that there remains a gap between the vision and what happens in reality. However, the process of implementation is under way, and many interviewees described their organisation as moving in the right direction. The difficulties of actually tackling community involvement were acknowledged, and issues raised included: the presence of other priorities which could knock community involvement off the agenda, lack of knowledge and experience, and difficulties in engaging hard-to-reach groups.

There is little doubt that the PCTs in Bradford are developing their capacity to support community involvement activity. The result is that there is growing dialogue with communities in localities and across the district. Mechanisms for community involvement are developing and being utilised. These new mechanisms include PCT decision-making groups with community and voluntary-sector representation, and local health forums open to the public. PCTs are also taking part in other forums, such as Neighbourhood Forums, Regeneration Boards, and Healthy Living Centre partnerships.

Despite growing links between community groups and the PCTs, there were differences in the extent to which community agendas were perceived to be influencing decision making. Although dialogue is taking place, those working in the PCTs acknowledged that at this stage communities are not yet routinely engaged in planning and decision making.

Learning about change

Building community involvement into mainstream health service business is new and presents numerous challenges, particularly given the rapidly changing policy context. The evaluation has helped facilitate reflection on the processes of change and enable learning to be documented. There is some understanding of the different factors that have influenced the work, which can be categorised into four groups: the national and district policy context, features of the PCTs as organisations, community capacity, and capacity in primary health care services. What is interesting is not so much the predictable barriers, such as lack of time or the huge agenda of change in the NHS, but the enabling factors which when present have facilitated the work. Good leadership on community involvement, a vision for the organisation, building infrastructure to support involvement, and good communication clearly help development of activity. Overall it appears that these enabling factors can militate against the negative effects of the huge agenda and workload. As one interviewee explained, it depends ultimately on how much value the organisation puts on community involvement. These findings have implications not only for the recruitment of key personnel but also indicate that time spent on organisational development and forming a shared vision provides a good basis for community involvement activity in health organisations.

The evaluation also found that the capacity of local communities to participate was influencing the pattern of activities undertaken. PCTs were reported to be more likely to engage with established groups, and there were concerns raised about reaching groups that have traditionally lacked a voice. Team members have been able to support groups who were new to involvement and in some cases offer practical help in terms of locating funding, premises or partners. The challenges of developing inclusive participatory processes remain, and these issues have been acknowledged by recent national proposals (DoH, 2001).

A specialist resource

Given the inexperience of community participation in primary care organisations, and evidence that previous activity has tended to been patchy (McIver, 1999; Brown, 2000), it has been suggested that PCTs could draw on expertise in community health councils, local authorities, community development agencies or other partners with similar expertise (Fisher and Gillam, 1999; Florin and Andersen, 2000). Indeed, a recent survey identified needs related to support and access to sources of expertise on involvement (Shepherd, 2001). In Bradford the model of support adopted has been one of a district team, with members attached to the PCTs. Findings indicate that PCTs do need to be able to draw on resources, in particular to develop links and contacts, and that the team's contribution to the development of community involvement has so far been significant. The nature of the project is about working in partnership with allies, within and outside the PCTs, and therefore it is not possible nor desirable to try to attribute the changes observed to the team alone.

One aspect of the team's success has been the speed at which it got going. HAZs were intended to act as drivers for change, and our findings demonstrate that the HAZ did enable the creation of a new resource that was able to rapidly engage in purposeful activities on the ground. The speed of transition seems to be related to a number of factors. These include: the team's clear understanding of the role and types of activities needed; the recruitment of team members who were very experienced in working with different communities, and in some cases had considerable local knowledge; and the presence of a good inter-agency infrastructure in the district, with other community development and regeneration initiatives in existence.

In addition, the model of a district team, as opposed to the involvement workers employed by separate PCTs, appears to have had some added value. Team members have been able to draw on the team for peer support, to share learning and to coordinate activity. In particular the team has enabled different models of practice to be shared and disseminated between PCTs. This way of working was called 'the Blue Peter model – here's one I made earlier' by the team manager. It appears to have prevented duplication of effort and helped implementation of activities.

What next?

The team was established with some degree of independence from the PCTs. There are now increasing tensions between maintaining a district approach and working in the context of the decentralisation agenda in the NHS, with PCTs wanting ownership of the work. As the funding of the team through the HAZ ends it will be taken up by the four PCTs, with each PCT employing a community involvement worker who will work from within their organisation. Issues of the location of the team raise more general questions about whether involvement workers are most effective when based in communities, local organisations or within a district infrastructure.

Primary care organisations in Bradford have responded to the community involvement agenda and developed capacity to begin to engage successfully with their local communities. There is a general perception among those interviewed that PCTs are keen to listen to, and incorporate, community views in their future planning. In the coming years it will be important to trace the impact of the early work and see whether it does bring benefits and improved services to local communities, and also whether participation deepens to include sustainable community–agency partnerships and community-initiated activity. This evaluation has focused on investigating organisational change, but there is another side to the story and gathering some community perceptions of involvement activity will be the next stage. Work has already been taking place in Bradford to adapt and develop a community involvement evaluation tool for organisations in the district, based on the Active Partners Framework (Yorkshire Forward, 2000).

A useful model

The evaluation has shown that it has been possible to use the opportunity provided by the HAZ to extend prior work in the district on community involvement. A specialist team was developed and has been able to act as a catalyst for activities, and a source of expertise and support for the newly formed PCGs/PCTs. The approach adopted in Bradford offers a useful model for implementing community involvement and translating strategic intentions into actions. The key features of this model are:

- focus on organisational development
- a capacity-building approach – enabling not substituting
- experienced community workers
- a resource within organisations
- a district team to aid coordination.

PCTs, alongside other health organisations, are currently having to respond to a strengthened patient and public involvement agenda. Community involvement workers, such as the Bradford HAZ Community Involvement Team, can potentially have a valuable role in helping PCTs implement a range of national involvement initiatives, such as the establishment of patient forums. In addition they can support PCTs in becoming active in local partnerships and initiatives such as Neighbourhood Renewal. In Bradford the continued funding of the work indicates that the PCTs recognise the value of having a specialist resource, and want to make community involvement part of their organisations' core work. In that sense Bradford HAZ has been successful in facilitating the leap from community involvement as innovative work on a 'wish list' to seeing changes in the mainstream.

References

Brown, I. (2000) 'Involving the public in general practice in an urban district: levels and type of activity and perceptions of obstacles', *Health and Social Care in the Community*, 8/4, 251–9.

DoH (2001) *Involving patients and the public in healthcare: a discussion document*, September, Department of Health.

Fawcett, B. (2000) 'Look, listen, learn', *Community Care*, 27 July–2 August, 24–5.

Fisher, B. and Gillam, S. (1999) 'Community development in the new NHS', *British Journal of General Practice*, 49, 428–30.

Florin, D. and Anderson, N. (2000) 'Public involvement: whose priority and whose responsibility?', *British Journal of Health Care Management*, 6/6, 258–61.

McIver, S. (1999) 'Public involvement in primary care: implications for primary care groups', *Nursing Times Research*, 4/4, 245–56.

NHS Executive (1999) *Patient and public involvement in the new NHS*, Department of Health, HSC 199/210.

Shepherd, M. (2001) 'Voice recognition', *Health Service Journal*, 15 February, 32–3.

Wilson, R. (1999) *Community involvement infrastructure in the Bradford district: soundings taken with 16 local organisations*, April, Bradford: Ruth Wilson Associates.

Yorkshire Forward (2000) *Active partners: benchmarking community participation in regeneration*, Leeds: Yorkshire Forward.

CHAPTER 3

Taking the risk to blossom: the Salford Social Entrepreneurs Programme

Chris Dabbs

> 'And the day came when the risk to remain tight in a bud was more painful than the risk it took to blossom.'
>
> Anaïs Nin

Introduction

The City of Salford lies within Greater Manchester, and includes both an inner-city heartland and several townships. All wards except one experience poor health, and in some cases major health inequalities, strongly associated with socioeconomic deprivation. The City was included in the large, first-wave Manchester, Salford and Trafford Health Action Zone, which had a strong commitment to the participation of local citizens, not only as groups and communities, but also as individuals.

The purpose of the Salford Social Entrepreneurs Programme – the first of its type in the United Kingdom – is to increase the confidence, capacity and skills of local people to tackle problems in their own communities through practical improvements. It has sought to do this by forming a cluster of five 'community sparkplugs' to work on projects in their own areas – for which they decided the form, nature and theme – within a full-time learning programme over one year.

The programme ran as a pilot from November 1999 to October 2000, funded by the Health Action Zone. It was jointly run by the School for Social Entrepreneurs (SSE) and Salford Community Health Council.

Lessons learnt

At the end of the programme the participants identified a range of personal and project achievements. They stated that the best things about the SSE were networks, visits, action learning, kudos and employment. In terms of areas for change, participants highlighted issues of mixing people with different levels of knowledge and experience, clarity of roles, and even more engagement with those working at 'grassroots' levels.

The processes for recruitment and selection of participants were crucial to the success of the programme. The almost completely oral and networking approach to this was very effective.

Self-esteem

The fundamental factor in the effectiveness of the Programme was the development of the self-confidence and self-esteem of all the participants. They particularly reflected on this regarding dealings with anyone in formal authority. Such development was supported by many factors, especially growing self-awareness and self-control, support and faith available, paid employment, raised status through association with a respected organisation, increasing resources of knowledge and practical successes in projects.

Personal development and learning

All the participants had felt very daunted by the programme at its beginning. This was coupled with an anxiety that the SSE was somehow going to change them against their will. This was not borne out. Participants became increasingly aware of their own personal development and learning over the year, and the different learning methods used suited all the participants. Individuals developed, however, in contrasting ways that created a challenge for the SSE. Those with the greatest experience of community activism had to 'chip away' at some of the 'armour' they had developed over many years. This was sometimes a slow and difficult process. Others with less experience blossomed at a significant rate, to a level where their 'overenthusiasm' had to be reined in a little.

Participants perceived in the programme an overemphasis on personal development and an imbalance against project development. There was truth in this in the earlier months, but experience suggests that it is very important to 'front-load' the personal development elements and confidence-building. This includes more emphasis on assertiveness, stress and time management, presentation skills, balancing work and home commitments, and psychological barriers to exploring outside existing knowledge and networks. Success in projects is partly related to personal development, especially in terms of self-esteem and self-confidence. The balance with project development can be reclaimed later in the programme.

A general resistance to writing things down (in which there was a notable lack of confidence) hampered the use of personal development plans. Gradually, however, this began to be overcome.

The programme enabled people to review and begin to adjust their individual approach, presentation and style. They became more focused and proactive. They also positively improved their approach to working in a group, and the impression they gave to 'expert witnesses' and visitors from outside. The development of self-confidence enabled individuals to make changes in their behaviours and attitudes.

Personal development supported individual achievements, not only in skills development and practical projects, but also in personal matters, such as remaining calm, losing weight, stopping smoking and becoming less dependent.

At the end of the year, participants stressed that, through the programme, they had learnt to organise their ideas and to present them in a variety of ways appropriate to the situation. They also learnt to negotiate, challenge and realise that 'no' does not have to be the final answer.

Project development

Initially seen as 'difficult' and not used much at home, the comment workbook *Opening the doors to third sector business planning* was latterly found more relevant and helpful, alongside exercises in the study sessions.

In the second half of the programme, when beginning to realise the significance of business plans, participants said that they would have liked the idea of business planning introduced earlier (although it was introduced on day one!).

Two things are clear from this experience. First, more emphasis and intensive work are required at the start of the programme on the need for and benefits of doing project development plans, while relating this more practically to individual projects. Second, throughout the programme, there needs to be focused work at both group and individual levels on project development during reviews and study days.

Engaging and influencing local people

A key learning point for all participants concerned getting the community actively involved from an early stage. One person found this easy to do, and offers of help were forthcoming. Another found that the community was interested to help but individuals were loath to take on parts of the project themselves. A third felt that people in her community seemed to want the project to happen, but were reluctant to participate.

Nevertheless, there were many examples of how the SSE projects prompted direct participation by other local people, such as becoming company directors, taking up courses such as bookkeeping and child care, and developing a better understanding of local government structures and procedures. The projects also changed some other local people on a personal level, with regard to their own self-confidence, for example.

Engaging other organisations

At times, projects did not develop as swiftly as participants wanted. This was, in part, due to difficulties experienced with individuals, cultures and structures within some statutory agencies. As the year progressed, however, projects secured help and support from a range of sources – community groups, housing associations and larger voluntary organisations, and local and regional statutory bodies.

Financial and practical support secured for projects included help with consultation, the services of a community architect, and support for negotiation of leases.

Learning by doing

'Learning by doing' is the fundamental principle of the SSE. Some members of the Supporters' Network did, however, express a concern that the programme might still be too intellectual, and might dampen spirit and instinct. They also recognised, however, that the programme is a guide to the process of 'getting there': there is no blueprint for success.

Participants were supported in their learning by having an action learning set – a 'priceless' opportunity for discussion – complementing the local support from the SSE coordinator and tutor and the personal mentors, all of whom were highly valued. Peer education with each other and with others on SSE programmes elsewhere in the United Kingdom also got high praise.

The programme faced a difficult balance between planning ahead and providing 'just-in-time' learning through the closer linking of programme topics to project demands. The School recognises that expert knowledge is of most value when directly relevant to current need to know. Approaches were developed to try to link more clearly – on a 'current need-to-know' basis – the experience of group activities, including the provision of expert knowledge, to individual and project development. This remained, however, an area of tension in itself because, in order to secure dates, it was necessary to book expert witnesses and visits as and when available, rather than more flexibly according to the learning needs of the group.

While inquiry and discussion of individual experience were taken up effectively from early in the programme, testing and applying lessons from this in projects were much slower. By the second quarter of the programme the action learning set facilitator concluded that 'there is continual progress ... [the participants] are learning from the actions they are taking'. On a less serious note, from their first study week in London the SSE group learnt to travel light, and expressed greater appreciation of some positive aspects of Salford, despite its shortcomings.

Throughout the year the main areas for application were written and verbal communication and presentation skills, and networking at different levels (including with politicians and larger organisations). Other fields included: creating and exploiting new opportunities, record keeping, and use of the media and presentations. Participants also stated that they gained better understandings of funding, research, statutory structures, and project development and implementation – including 'greater awareness of sustainability issues'.

Study days, study weeks, visits and expert witnesses

Study days

Participants' responses to study days remained equally divided through the year. Half found them mainly enjoyable, informative and one of the best parts of the programme. Those with more experience felt that too long was spent on subjects of which they were already aware.

Study weeks

The mixing of local and national programme participants at the study weeks in London was not a success. The content and style of any such mixing must be considered very carefully to make sure that they meet the needs of both styles of programme. It is likely that the best topics for content are those that deal with interpersonal issues, rather than those of social policy or 'hard' business planning skills.

Visits

Although initially there were concerns that time spent on visits took participants away from their project development, they were soon cited as one of the best parts of the whole programme, without which the participants would not have made them.

'Expert witnesses'

All the participants valued the opportunities to meet and question 'expert witnesses'. Most were described as 'brilliant' and 'inspiring'. Especially useful was the opportunity to ask specific questions and develop personal contacts. In particular, the experts offered hope and inspiration from their proven track records.

Networking

One of the most positive aspects of the programme was the increased possibility of new contacts and networks for participants, not only in the present, but also for the future.

Area initiatives and regeneration programmes

During the year, participants developed not only their local networks but also links with local regeneration programmes, especially the Single Regeneration Budget and the city council's community strategy. They found it difficult, however, to establish many links with the Health Action Zone. This was mainly because of its refocusing in Salford towards a single development site that did not include the participants' communities. There were, however, contacts made with the two primary care groups and their health improvement programmes.

Outside Salford

Participants forged new links and partners outside Salford throughout the year. This was, however, a slower process than at local level. There remained evidence of some anxiety (although declining) about expanding and broadening networks, especially outside each person's locality, which suggests a need to provide more support and encouragement in this area (though one person stated that some of the information might not be relevant in the first year).

Skills and training

During the year, participants developed and applied their skills from a wide range of training and development opportunities. Some of these were informal, while others were accredited or led to qualifications such as NVQs. The participants all developed skills in areas such as project, time and resource management; written and verbal communication; and negotiation.

Participants were reassured about the approach to learning – not least that training and development are not one and the same. There was then a marked change in their approach, with less emphasis on attending training courses and more on broader development opportunities. The amount of formal training reduced significantly, especially as projects began to develop. This reflected a growing general understanding that the programme was about learning rather than teaching. Reassurance about this seems to have reduced the use of the 'comfort blanket' of training courses.

Participants increasingly realised the relevance of business skills such as planning. There was a need to repeat work on this throughout the programme to help individuals become accustomed to this approach, and to await the time at which each realised its practical relevance. Nevertheless, all participants retained some resistance to writing, administration and paper-based work. With one exception (a very task-centred person), they found it difficult to work individually on their ideas and obviously much preferred talking through the subjects as a group. Nevertheless, there was a very apparent increase over the year in the quality of written plans, proposals and strategies produced.

Programme management

It was recognised from early on that the programme – as a national pilot – had no direct precedents. It therefore inevitably 'had teeting problems, but overall it's been good'.

Length of the programme

Several people – supporters, participants and staff – questioned the length of the programme. Is 12 months long enough for people and projects to sufficiently establish themselves, or was the SSE not ensuring that they focus on things hard enough to secure their personal situation by month 13? The actual development of individuals and projects suggests, however, that 12 months may be adequate, given the right level of motivation and support, and may avoid creating overdependence.

Programme arrangements

The various elements of the programme enabled many potential points of contact and learning for the participants. There is, however, a need for greater integration between the 'hard' business skills of the programme – sometimes a more formal learning process – and the softer skills of confidence building, assertiveness and negotiation.

Practical challenges

There were some practical problems at the start of the programme. For example, participants did not enjoy travelling to study days, while the usefulness of the electronic communication offered was only realised towards the end of the programme. The national e-learning seminar had limited success, with only some participants making significant contributions to the discussion, although for some this was their first major attempt to use electronic communication.

Staff recruitment and support

The recruitment criteria and payment rates for local staff are important. Staff should have the range and complexity of skills needed to deliver the programme and to support participants with complex learning and support needs.

While local staff became clearer about their individual roles and functions, there remained a lack of clarity about who was responsible for which decisions at national level. Consequently, the decision-making process was somewhat drawn out or ad hoc. The national coordinator had to develop policy and procedures 'on the hoof' as local circumstances arose. With the benefit of the Salford experience, these are now in place and can be applied to future programmes.

The amount of support needed by both local and national staff on the programme was underestimated. The actual lead-in time for the programme was appropriate, but allocations for the frequency and intensity of support during the lead-in and delivery of the programme needed to be reassessed.

Assessing effectiveness

A main concern of the Supporters' Network was assessing the effectiveness of the programme. This implied clarifying the desired goals and outcomes in order to define the measures of success. This was achieved through the development process that produced the theory of change (see Table 3.1). It was suggested that the SSE should do a cost–benefit analysis of the programme to demonstrate its cost-effectiveness.

Despite these challenges, one supporter wrote: 'In my view, the scheme is excellent value for money and a worthwhile investment for the [Health Action Zone]'.

Table 3.1 Salford Social Entrepreneurs Programme: theory of change

Context/problem	Rationale/strategy	Assumptions	Intervention	Expected consequences	Assumptions
• Problems in communities	• To increase the confidence, capacity, knowledge and skills of local people to tackle the problems of their own communities	• People learn best by taking action	• Employ local people as community entrepreneurs	• Increased self-confidence, self-esteem and status of social entrepreneurs	• Appropriate people recruited to the programme
• School for Social Entrepreneurs		• Other practitioners with a track record provide the most valuable material	• Enable development of mutual support between social entrepreneurs	• Other local people take up new opportunities	• The programme addresses individual needs
• Health Action Zone		• Expert knowledge is of most value when directly relevant to the current need-to-know	• Provide learning opportunities (e.g. expert witnesses, visits, action learning)	• Social entrepreneurs have broader vision and adopt new, more effective approaches to problem-solving	• The programme is appropriate to individual social entrepreneur's needs
• Lack of accessible/ appropriate educational and other opportunities and resources	• To change the attitude, approach and behaviour of local people to problems and finding solutions	• Personal development increases confidence	• Provide support, mentoring and contacts for project development	• Greater capacity, knowledge and skills to address issues	• The programme is responsive, flexible and delivered at an appropriate time
• Insufficient resources for community action	• To give local people access to local, regional and national (support) networks	• Increased confidence and knowledge are empowering and lead to action	• Provide access to new contacts and networks	• Access to a wider range of contacts and networks	
• Lack of resources to support individual 'community sparkplugs'	• To attain a new perspective on challenging social exclusion	• People can learn much from their peers	• Introduce people to new and challenging experiences and ideas	• Increased capacity for learning	
		• Self-awareness enables people to use talents, make choices and solve problems better		• Increased control by local people to improve their own wellbeing	
		• Individuals have different learning needs and learn in different ways		• Greater knowledge about how to support and develop social entrepreneurs	
		• Communities can benefit from the actions of community entrepreneurs			

The future

The participants

All the participants had an ever-present concern about their future after the end of the SSE Programme. There was particular anxiety about possibly returning from paid work to state benefits. The participants felt that support and guidance on this should have been addressed even earlier than it was, right from the start of the year.

Support and guidance were offered during the year to plan and to obtain the resources to achieve a secure way forward. Work was done to support participants to develop and implement exit strategies. It was impressive that the aims of participants and their projects became much more tightly focused in the second half of the year, including maintaining and developing their networks.

Some participants created more positive positions for themselves than others. All of them had to be supported and encouraged to push harder to achieve this, while recognising that ultimately the responsibility is theirs.

Each of the participants who joined the SSE not only achieved significant personal development from the start of the Salford Programme, but also made great progress with their projects. At the end of the year the participants were reminded that they had expressed great anxiety in around month 8 of the programme about what would happen at its end. Some had felt that the SSE had a responsibility to provide ongoing support and help. The entire group now felt less anxious. They had greater confidence that they would be able to continue with their projects without a structured programme and, as part of the network of SSE fellows, would be able to use the School to get the help they might need. They felt that this might include: a continued relationship with staff and other SSE Fellows, advice and guidance, development of information and communication technology skills, and a review of progress in two to three years' time.

The SSE and social entrepreneurship in Salford and the Health Action Zone

In 2001, as a result of the pilot programme, the SSE successfully secured investment to establish a Salford School for Social Entrepreneurs. This complemented Millennium Awards for up to seven Salford people to participate in the second Salford SSE Programme in 2002.

The SSE in Salford has engaged with many local agencies both to develop effective support for and to reduce hindrances to social and community entrepreneurs in the City. A longer-term approach and strong infrastructure are essential if the role of social entrepreneurship is to achieve its maximum benefit. Links with the Salford Partnership and into the Salford Community Plan are vital, especially on both social inclusion and economic development. Joint work by the SSE with the Community Action Network and Salford Community Venture has led to initial developments to support the social economy in Salford.

The SSE looks forward to continued work with the Health Action Zone to develop the latter's commitment 'to evaluate the School for Social Entrepreneurs and [to try] to secure long term funding if it is shown to be successful'. Links into local strategic partnerships and approaches to neighbourhood renewal will be particularly important if the lessons from the pilot SSE programme in Salford are to be mainstreamed and to be extended into other areas.

The SSE and social entrepreneurship in North-West England

Regionally, the SSE has continued its collaboration with the Community Action Network and the Scarman Trust. The lessons from the pilot SSE Programme in Salford have informed the development of a regional approach to support social enterprise, with support from the North West Development Agency.

The SSE and social entrepreneurship in the United Kingdom

The experience of the Salford SSE pilot programme has also informed and influenced the approaches to small businesses in deprived communities by the Bank of England and HM Treasury, and the government's National Strategy for Neighbourhood Renewal.

Learning from the lessons of the pilot local programme in Salford, SSE programmes have already been established in Belfast and Glasgow. More were established in 2001 in several urban and rural locations across England.

The SSE experience in Salford informed the development of the model for the work of unLTD (the National Foundation for Social Entrepreneurs) and its work to support social and community entrepreneurs at different levels across the regions and nations within the United Kingdom. This should continue in perpetuity and make social entrepreneurship a permanent feature in the social and economic landscape.

A participant's final thought

This course has been to me an experience of a lifetime and I think there should be more money available for more activists to go on the course. The world would be a better place for all of us. This is what communities lack – *support* and *communication*. The skills I have gained while on the programme I will pass on to my community. Invest in the School for Social Entrepreneurs Programme: 'you won't be sorry'.

2 December 2001

Conclusions

The SSE approach to supporting individuals as 'community sparkplugs' proved largely successful in terms of both personal and project development. The longer-term impact on the health and wellbeing of local populations remains to be seen, but the signs are promising. Backing individuals has value, but as a complement rather than a competitor to community-based approaches.

CHAPTER 4

The reality of participatory research and public involvement

Jane Sharpe, Janet Bostock, Jean Bell and Judith Brown

Introduction

In this chapter we describe the community survey we supported in order to inform the development of a Community and Training Centre that was being built in Blyth, south-east Northumberland. We discuss the background to the work undertaken, the participatory methods used, the impact the survey had on public involvement in the community, and the benefits, challenges and lessons to be learnt from this approach to community needs assessment.

Background

The wards of Cowpen and Kitty Brewster are situated in Blyth, south-east Northumberland. Since the decline of local industries such as coal mining and shipbuilding they have now been targeted as priority wards eligible for European funding due to their high levels of deprivation. Unemployment is high, and low levels of car ownership and poor public transport services restrict residents' ability to access jobs and training opportunities in other parts of the region. Further to this, the two wards have a very high proportion of people classified as being long-term sick or disabled, and Kitty Brewster has a standard mortality rate of 316, over three times the national average.

Cowpen and Kitty Brewster Community Association hoped to address some of the needs of the community in their plans for a Community and Training Centre. The centre was being built at the time this research was being carried out. The new facility contains several multipurpose training rooms, a training kitchen and a multi-activity sports area.

There was a recent history of active public involvement and partnership working in the area, which included:

• a local strategy for public involvement

- active community and economic development workers employed by the district council
- community involvement work with the Northumberland Health Action Zone and the receipt of a small HAZ grant to promote public involvement
- a number of energetic voluntary community activists on the estate.

The objectives of the research were:

1 to enable community centre volunteers to understand local needs for the development of the centre
2 to engage local people in the centre's activities
3 to enable local people to influence the design, delivery and follow-up to the research
4 to highlight the needs of individuals and groups who might be excluded from initial enquiries by accessing voluntary and community groups and mental health and primary care service users.

In summary, the research process aimed to promote public involvement.

Method

Figure 4.1 presents the stages of the research and shows how the process was cyclical.

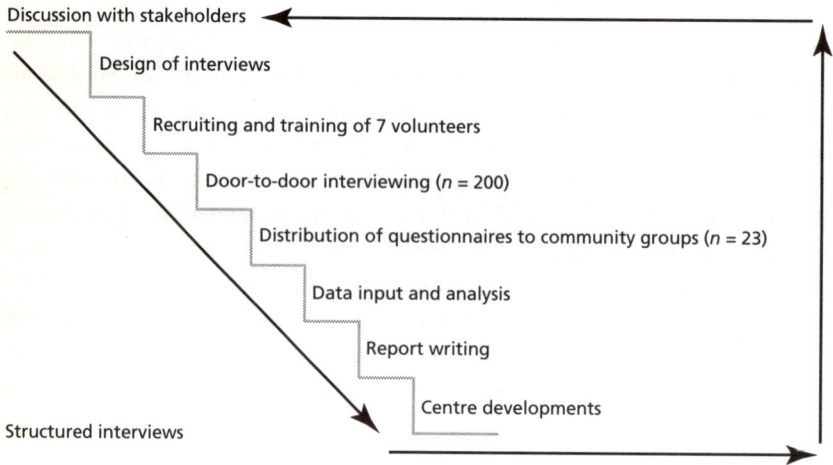

Discussion with stakeholders

Design of interviews

Recruiting and training of 7 volunteers

Door-to-door interviewing (*n* = 200)

Distribution of questionnaires to community groups (*n* = 23)

Data input and analysis

Report writing

Centre developments

Structured interviews

Figure 4.1: The research process

The planning group consisted of volunteers from the community association, a community worker, a community psychologist and a research assistant. We decided that the information would be collected via structured door-to-door interviews because we wanted to meet people face-to-face and to gain a substantial proportion of local views. We did not consider that random or representative sampling was possible in the timescale. The planning group determined the content of the interviews, which were divided into five sections relating to different planned/possible community projects.

Questions asked in the survey

Community activities

The first part of the survey investigated whether or not people would become involved in certain planned or suggested courses and activities, or use resources in the centre. Further ideas were also sought from the respondents themselves.

Community transport

From previous community appraisals, it was evident that access around the two wards was difficult for many people. The second part of the survey sought to highlight the difficulties of travelling and to determine the support for community transport schemes, including a community bus with subsidised fares.

Money

Anecdotal evidence suggested that many people in the community had problems opening a bank account because of the documentation and starting sum needed. This was identified as a barrier to work, because if people had no bank account, they had nowhere to cash a pay cheque. A suggested solution to this problem was to have a bank owned by the community, where everyone banked their cheques and could receive money at the end of the week. The collective interest would be used for community projects.

Rather than asking people sensitive questions regarding whether they had problems opening accounts or whether they would use the bank, people were asked if they thought such a system would work and whether 'they or *anyone they knew*' would use it.

Sense of community

Increasing evidence shows that social cohesion is critical for societies to prosper economically and for development to be sustainable. Levels of social cohesion have also been linked with health (Campbell and Jovchelovitch, 2000). What was termed 'community spirit' or 'a sense of community' in the survey was drawing on the concept of social capital. Social capital is described as a community resource that is formed from social interactions and networks, based on the principles of trust, reciprocal relationships and community participation for mutual benefit (Putnam, 1993). It was envisaged that a sense of community would be enhanced by people's use of the centre.

The questionnaire enabled the collection of qualitative data on people's opinions about 'a sense of community'. Questions about people's friends and family, reciprocal help and support were also used to assess people's needs.

Identifying volunteers and specific needs

The steering group suggested that a befriending scheme might be set up to increase the level of volunteering in the area while meeting specific needs of individuals. It would work like a dating service, putting people in need in touch with people with time on their hands and skills to offer. People were asked whether they would like to become more involved in this or in any other projects at the centre.

Volunteer recruitment, training and management

To attract volunteers to the project, adverts were placed in community buildings and local shops stating that people over the age of 16 were required to do market research for one week in August. Seven volunteers were recruited, mainly through knowing people involved in the centre. A training day in research methods was held for the volunteers, led by a number of people, including a representative of a mental health user organisation who was experienced in research. The training included background information on the project; practical experience of using the questionnaire; interview techniques; ethical and safety issues; and discussion of the streets to cover.

In the four days following the training, 200 interviews were completed in a door-to-door survey. Lunch was provided daily, which was a good way to get people together for feedback and support in the middle of the day, and to hand in data. The interviewers worked in pairs, each with a different area to cover highlighted on their maps. At the end of the week, all the volunteers received a gift and a certificate. One interviewer who was enthusiastic about the project and good at engaging with people on the street stayed on another week to help with the next stage of the research.

Visiting community groups and targeting people who were harder to reach

Interviewers were asked to write down ideas of groups to contact, and places to go to get a wider sample and to reach people who would not be reached in a door-to-door survey. Questionnaires and flyers inviting people to take part in the research were then dropped off in these places. The community and voluntary organisations were willing distributors.

It was thought that by going through the mental health services and medical centres in Blyth, people would be reached who were socially isolated, and who were most likely to be in need of the services and facilities in the centre.

Data input and analysis

Most of the spreadsheet data-entry was done by a woman on a work placement at the community centre. Although she had used computers a lot as an administrative assistant, she had no research experience, and setting up the spreadsheet and inputting the initial data were quite time-consuming.

As well as the spreadsheet for recording the responses to the questions, the names and addresses of the people who had expressed interest in getting more involved in the community projects were recorded on a database.

Results of the survey

Suggestions for use of the centre

- Most people interviewed said they would be most likely to use the centre in the evening rather than the daytime. There was a lot of interest in sports and arts activities, particularly self-defence (35%), football (31%), painting and photography.
- Advice and information services were popular, as well as different courses, especially computer skills (over 50%).
- Many people saw the need for activities for young people.

Community transport

- About half the people interviewed used the bus regularly.

- Difficulties about using public transport were expressed, the main one being cost.
- A majority of respondents (78%) said they would use a community bus.

Money

- Although about a third of the sample said they or someone they knew would use a community bank, people were generally not sure about whether the idea would work.
- A third of people interviewed said they would welcome support/advice on money matters.

Sense of community

- People had different ideas about what they thought a sense of community was, but most people did not answer the question. Those who did answer indicated that it was very important.
- Different ways in which a greater sense of community could be created in the area were suggested. The most frequent response was ensuring that young people and children had something to do.
- Questions about the contact people had with their friends and family indicated that most people had good support networks. Informal relationships were seen as more important as a source of help and advice than professional relationships.

Identifying volunteers and specific needs

- There was considerable support for a befriending service (84% thought it was a 'good idea').
- The survey identified 42 people who said they had a skill to offer the service and 21 people who said they could benefit from the service.
- The names and addresses of these people were noted, as well as those of people who said they would like to get more involved.
- Problems people had with using the centre were identified, e.g. transport, lack of time.
- Over half the sample said that they would like to receive more information on what was happening in the area.

The impact of the survey on developments at the centre

Continued reference was made to the opinions of community members and the results of the survey in the planning of the centre. Some of the popular suggestions from the survey were already happening at the centre: for example, a karate club was using the centre weekly, and a five-aside football league was being established. The training kitchen was completed and courses started in collaboration with the local further education college. Also on offer were history, art and computer courses, which proved to be popular in the survey, as well as youth activities.

The survey showed that there was a need for information and advice on health, employment and benefits issues. The centre responded to this need by having information leaflets and job advertisements (faxed from the Jobcentre) in the foyer, and by inviting agencies such as the Careers Service into the centre for a regular slot. There was also work done with other agencies regarding the issues of community banking and community transport. Meetings were held with the Community Federation about buying a community bus, and a local credit union expressed interested in having one of its satellites in the centre.

The results of the survey were also used for bids for government money through the Neighbourhood Management Structure and the 'Neighbours with Know-how' schemes.

Engaging people in public involvement through the survey

The survey contacted 223 people, either through interviews or questionnaires. This represented 6% of the population. The questionnaires were distributed in 19 projects/centres. Revisiting them a few weeks later we found there to be few responses in the boxes provided, although several had been returned to the centre. As well as an information gathering exercise, this research was useful as part of the promotion of the centre and awareness-raising about community projects. Workers at the centre followed up a list of people who said they would be interested in specific projects, and some of these started running groups according to their own interests (for example a fishing club).

Discussion

The Cowpen Community Survey illustrates how participatory action research can be used to develop questions to be addressed; devise methods of generating information; collect and collate information; analyse and interpret the information; and act on it in order to effect change. It is a 'research approach that consists of the maximum participation of stakeholders, those whose lives are affected by the problem under study, in the systematic collection and analysis of infor-

Table 4.1 Community involvement and participative action research

Level of involvement	Type of involvement	Examples
Very low	Receives information	Community members received information about the centre
Low	Consultation	Community members were interviewed
Medium	Partnership	Community researchers in partnership with centre and other facilitators
High	Delegated control	Volunteers ran projects as a result of doing the survey
Very high	Has control	The volunteer coordinator at the centre controlled the resources for the project

mation for the purpose of taking action and making change' (Nelson et al., 1998, 885). In terms of the definitions of community participation forwarded by Brotchie (1994) and Brager and Specht (1973), the research enabled different groups to be involved to different extents (see Table 4.1).

Undertaking participatory research

The methodology used was successful in meeting the first three objectives of this work, which were to engage local residents and stakeholders in the research and in the developments of the Community and Training Centre. The key aspects of this were as follows.

Control by local people

The remit for the survey was initiated by people living in this area, rather than by professionals or academic interests. Active, shared decision-making occurred during all the phases of the research – defining the issues to investigate, writing up reports, and disseminating and acting on the findings.

Collaborative and methodological issues

Methodological dilemmas were an ongoing consideration. Collaboration was not always a comfortable experience for researchers who are accustomed to more rigorously organised research designs, particularly with regard to sampling procedures. There was considerable opportunity for mutual and ongoing learning. For instance, we recognise now that the time constraints should have been altered so that piloting the interview schedules was more thorough. One of the more challenging issues in this research was the number of people involved. This meant that it was difficult to standardise data collection, thus affecting its reliability. Also, one person coded the raw data onto the spreadsheet while another analysed and presented the data. Rigorous methodology was not the priority for this survey; rather, it was more important to talk to as many local people as possible. However, more care could have been taken to plan the sample of people questioned, by selecting which streets to cover in a more logical way and recording non-respondents.

Practical issues

The research was coordinated from a building close to where the Community and Training Centre was being built, and the circumstances for the training and discussions were often chaotic and unpredictable – e.g. interruptions from loud drilling or queries about the new site.

Engaging community researchers

The collaboration between people with different knowledge and skills enabled rich and locally meaningful data to be generated. Engaging community interviewers brought a number of benefits. First they knew the geographical area, and second they often appeared to know people and gain more information than a stranger would have done. Some of them said they learnt new skills and gained confidence as a result of participating. All of the community interviewers for this study were unemployed at the time, with a history of temporary work and few qualifications. All but one said that they had enjoyed the project and would do it again. Some said they would like to get a job doing something similar, and others became interested in voluntary work at the centre and training in community work. However, most have lost contact with the centre now, and their involvement might have been sustained if they had been able to participate earlier in the project, for example, designing the questionnaires, and then helping to analyse the data. In this way they would have had a greater sense of ownership of the project, and would have learnt more skills.

A disadvantage of employing local people is that those participating in the research may feel uncomfortable sharing sensitive information with people they know socially. This may have been particularly true of the questions relating to money. This approach to community research may therefore be inappropriate for certain issues.

Practical outcomes

The research yielded practical outcomes that were useful to the community and enabled the better use of this community resource. It informed decisions, actions and policies. For instance, one of the interviewees was inspired to set up activities for young people in the area as a result of the interview.

Ongoing engagement with the public

The undertaking of the research enabled an outgoing approach to engaging the public. This remains a key aspect of the Community and Training Centre's work. For example, the current questionnaire in circulation from the centre is concerned with the housing and neighbourhood difficulties on the estate, with a view to resolving them with the council. The centre has become established in the community as a valuable, accessible resource, and has become an example of best practice for public involvement in the North East Assembly's Voice for the Region project.

Research process

The process of research such as this is important, and we sought to ensure that it was supportive, interesting and as pleasurable as possible. The volunteer on the Community Association who initiated the research, herself a member of the community, had most of the control of the resources throughout the project. The benefits for her were that she consolidated her authority and experience (she later became centre manager). She has also co-written a paper to enable others to conduct community surveys. The benefits for the project were that she lived in the area and was well informed about the issues, needs and culture, so could advise the other partners on methodology. In the long term, she was able to implement the findings of the research and involve more local people.

How effective was this participatory research in engaging marginalised or excluded individuals or groups?

The extent to which the engagement of those who were marginalised, socially isolated or usually excluded was achieved in the survey was not easily measured. From the results it seems that most of the sample had had some social contact, as 91% had seen someone in their family in the past week and 91% had talked to a friend. It would have been useful to include further questions about people's participation in social and community activity.

A positive outcome of the research was that staff (including Community Service Volunteers, social services, the Jobcentre and the Community Mental Health Team) contacted during the distribution of questionnaires to their clients made enquiries about activities at the centre. A strong link has been made between the Community and Training Centre and a nearby day service for people with enduring mental health problems. In addition, one of the trainers for the community interviewers was from a mental health service user organisation. One person who was referred to the centre from the Jobcentre to do voluntary work in the garden now volunteers there on a full-time basis. Through his involvement with people at the centre, his confidence is improving, and he comes across as less anxious and depressed. He has received help with welfare benefits and has been helped to access GP services, which has resulted in his being referred to a hand specialist. Following on from the survey there was a successful meeting at the centre about 'promoting user voices', which enabled an exchange of information and experiences from a number of user groups in the area. Continuous work with the centre staff and local people is required in order to ensure that this resource is used by those who most need opportunities for friendship and activity.

Conclusion

We suggest that participative community research is potentially a means of sharing expertise and experience in order to promote various forms of community involvement (which includes providing information, offering consultation, and enabling control and influence). In this project, systematic information was generated which had validity for the community involved. This collaborative work required cooperation between partners, funding for materials and volunteer expenses, and a proactive, flexible approach from those involved.

References

Brager, G. and Specht, H. (1973) *Community organizing*, New York: Columbia University Press.

Brotchie, J. (1994) *Managing social service delivery: responding to customers*, Oxford: Oxford University Press.

Campbell, C. and Jovchelovitch, S. (2000) 'Health, community and development: towards a social psychology of participation', *Journal of Community and Applied Social Psychology*, 10, 225–70.

Nelson, G., Ochocka, J., Griffin, K. and Lord, J. (1998) '"Nothing about me, without me": participatory action research with self-help/mutual aid organizations for psychiatric consumer/survivors', *American Journal of Community Psychology*, 26/6, 881–912.

Putnam, R. (1993) *Making democracy work*, New Jersey: Princeton University Press.

CHAPTER 5

Implicitly good – good for whom? A review of employing community evaluators

Sandra Squires and Michael Clark

Introduction

Wolverhampton was granted Health Action Zone status in 1999. From its inception, there was a commitment from partners in health, social care and community organisations to learn from the projects in the six workstreams. This was vital for the work to inform mainstream service development in the future. Hence, an Evaluation Network Group (ENG)[1] was convened to coordinate a variety of evaluation activities and reporting.

One explicit aspect of the evaluation strategy was to assess how projects were working for local people. As with most evaluation work, the group was faced with a variety of audiences for its findings and credibility had to be gained in all their eyes. In keeping with the spirit of the HAZ, namely being innovative, building local capacity and increasing participation, the ENG sought to marry this with evaluation requirements of methodological rigour, trained personnel and community orientation.

One of the key evaluation projects of the group was the community evaluator initiative. The idea of local people being involved in regeneration-oriented evaluation is not new, but is gaining national credibility. The assumption is that local people know best about local needs and can act as 'honest brokers' between these needs and organisational development. This paper outlines the project and its progress towards meeting three broad objectives of evaluation, increasing employment opportunities for job seekers and public participation.

---

[1] Comprising HAZ coordinator, workstream leads, external consultant from the university, research and development coordinator, Wolverhampton Health Care Trust, assistant director of public health and the senior evaluator.

Early steps

Initial discussions aimed to give direction to the loosely defined idea of assessing public perception of HAZ services. The employment workstream had experience of establishing intermediate labour markets (ILMs), the aim of which is to provide a bridge back into work for those most marginalised from the labour market. The exact nature of the work is not important. Of more importance is that the employees have appropriate training and support, have a worthwhile employment experience and are better equipped to find longer-term employment. This fitted a key HAZ aim and hence became a core objective of this project.

Underpinning assumptions

The ENG embarked on a path to create a community evaluation ILM. Combining HAZ and ILM philosophies gave the project certain ideological assumptions. These were:

1 there were local, long-term unemployed people, of a particular profile, who would be interested in this kind of work
2 these people could undertake the work with a certain level of support
3 employing people to do this kind of work through the ILM and on the minimum wage was a fair thing to do
4 worthwhile, respect-worthy evaluation could be produced
5 the project would benefit recruits in terms of their longer-term employment opportunities
6 it would provide a cheaper way of undertaking evaluation than contracting external evaluators
7 employing community evaluators would aid the ENG by demonstrating its commitment to the HAZ values of innovation, community involvement and addressing inequalities
8 having community evaluators would add something to the evaluation that would otherwise be missed by having external evaluators. This assumption itself had two dimensions:
   – their 'localness' and coming from outside the statutory organisations meant they had unique and valuable perspectives to contribute
   – being local afforded them privileged access to frank and sincere opinions of HAZ service users
9 community evaluators and the outcomes of their work had the potential to act as honest brokers between communities and organisational development; if found to work, this model could offer one avenue to implement government policy of developing more client-centred services through increasing public participation in decision making

10 the project could be used as a first step in a wider programme of community engagement and capacity building.

With hindsight it is clearer that these assumptions were largely implicit in the project. From the outset there was a general feeling among the ENG of its being a 'good' thing to do, but, if pressed, the different members of the group would probably have provided different criteria regarding why this was the case. This vagueness has, perhaps surprisingly, been one of the strengths contributing to the project's successful outcomes, though there were consequences.

Establishing the initiative

The employment workstream took responsibility for seeking funding from the Single Regeneration Budget 4 and the European Social Fund (contributing 45% of the minimum wage). Pulling together the cocktail of funding and conditions required to run an ILM is an involved task. The total cost was £72,412, with the HAZ contributing £25,553. The key element missing from these costs is that of the time of the HAZ senior evaluator.

While an accredited training programme was delivered, the ENG began to define in more specific terms the role of the evaluators. The debate considered such issues as the extent to which they would be employed as 'market researchers', implementing set questionnaires devised by the ENG, or as independent evaluators, with the scope to define and own their work, and whether the focus should be geographic or project-based.

It was decided that a project-based approach would be of most benefit to the HAZ through its impact on local policy development. The workstream leads each identified two projects they would like to be evaluated. The evaluators chose from this list. Although two chose the same (large) project and this meant fewer projects would be evaluated than hoped for, it was agreed that the evaluators could work side by side.

Another consideration was the timescale for the project. Figure 5.1 represents the envisaged timeline for the initiative, which did not alter a great deal during implementation. The chief change was the number of projects evaluated within six months. In part this was a question of feasibility, especially given the tension between short-term contracts and seeking employment. Also, some of the projects chosen by the evaluators were more detailed than initially envisaged and required the full six months to complete. Two other factors were the varied skill levels of recruits and a management style which imposed few deadlines.

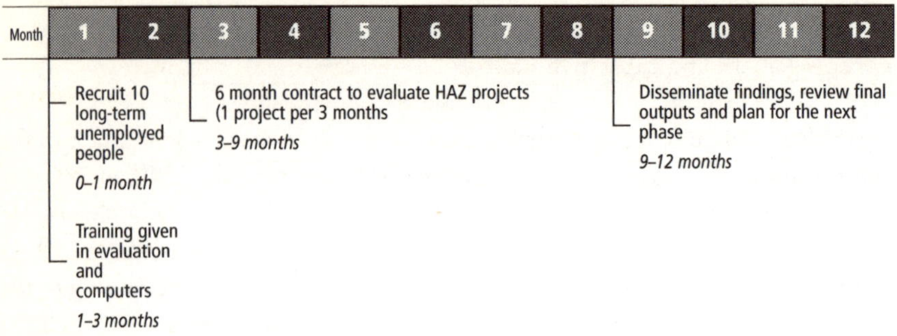

Month	1	2	3	4	5	6	7	8	9	10	11	12

Recruit 10
long-term
unemployed
people

0–1 month

Training given
in evaluation
and
computers

1–3 months

6 month contract to evaluate HAZ projects
(1 project per 3 months)

3–9 months

Disseminate findings, review final
outputs and plan for the next
phase

9–12 months

Figure 5.1: Initial timeline for the community evaluator project

Introducing the community evaluators

Ten participants began the training in community research and evaluation skills. Only eight actually started the work, as two dropped out for personal reasons in the first week of training. The discussion below is based on exit interviews with the eight who undertook evaluation work.

The employment workstream sought to recruit to the project through promotional days, adverts in the local paper and vacancies posted with the Jobcentre. There was the tacit expectation that the job seekers coming forward for interview would have low educational achievement and have been unemployed for some time. In reality this was not so. In fact the list of interviewees was almost a graduation roll call – five had degrees, two had undertaken two years of their degree course (but not completed them for various reasons), and another was a school leaver having just finished her A levels. Their employment status before starting as community evaluators was also not as expected: only two (both male) had been unemployed for more than six months, and five had been homebuilders and were seeking to move into paid employment (see Table 5.1).

It is of note that the women returners were not recruited through the Jobcentres, but came via promotional/recruitment fairs, notice boards and newspaper advertisements. Nobody found his or her way through local community groups.

Table 5.1 Employment history of the community evaluators before the project

Employment status before starting	Level of seeking work
Student, female (1)	Actively seeking work (4)
Home career, not registered unemployed, female (4)	Keeping an eye out for something interesting (4)
Home career, less than 6 months unemployed, female (1)	
Long-term unemployed, male (2)	

Table 5.2 Social profile of the eight community evaluators

	Heritage		
Female : male	Indian subcontinent	English	Irish
6:2	5	2	1

Once again, the power of hindsight illuminates an area that was left too implicit in the planning of the project. Perhaps the idea of the work created the impression in the heads of potential recruits and staff in Jobcentres that people of particular qualifications and/or experience would be required. This may have meant that the long-term unemployed people that the ENG was implicitly expecting were deterred from applying. The result, however, perhaps worked to the benefit of the project. The generally high qualification levels of the recruits may have reduced the amount of direct supervision required and helped to ensure a high level of final reporting. This, however, is an untested assumption and an area that we would like to explore further when extending the work of community evaluation.

The social profile of the eight community evaluators is interesting (see Table 5.2). In particular, the project was very successful in attracting from the Asian communities, although it is noticeable that there were no African-Caribbean recruits. Their reports can be viewed on their web page, found at www.healthactionzone.co.uk.

Lessons learnt

Throughout the course of the project a variety of lessons have been learnt that put us in good stead to extend community evaluation in Wolverhampton. Here we would like to review those lessons before further discussing the implicit assumptions behind the project.

Support

The first lesson is that support has been key to the success of the initiative and has taken many guises. Initially a supportive environment was required to deliver training to a group with diverse educational achievements, mixed work experience and various states of preparedness to re-engage with the working world.

The second element of the supportive environment was that of the peer support the evaluators gave to themselves. Bonds forged during training were sustained at work. This led to the third essential support element: during the evaluation work a weekly meeting of the evaluators, the project manager and occasional guest speakers was held to discuss the work, and contact outside this two-hour meeting was made available by an open-door policy. This allowed the evaluators to discuss specific issues with the manager.

The evaluators valued this support, but there were lessons to be learnt. While five of the group found the weekly meetings useful, two felt that they were too unstructured, and neither gained nor contributed much. It might have been better value to improve the programme of invited guests and to have had some structured tutorials covering gaps identified in the training, especially with regard to report writing.

A computer technician provided support with databases and data analysis. This enabled the evaluators to undertake quantitative analysis of their work and present graphic displays of their data. These visuals gave added professionalism and emphasis to their reports.

In the background to this immediate support was that of the ENG itself. The whole group was not directly involved in the evaluations once they were under way. Key people in the group were, however, involved in reviewing the planned evaluations. The persuasive argument that each evaluator seeks to collect the same socioeconomic data was helpful in the long run. All the community evaluators were required to ask the postcode, age, ethnic background and occupation (of interviewee or relevant household member) of all service users surveyed. This has been illuminating, as we can summarise who the beneficiaries of the HAZ projects have been. The socioeconomic data from each project has been analysed and an aggregate profile of all service users surveyed has been produced by the evaluators themselves.

One further aspect of support relating to the community evaluators was their generosity of spirit in supporting an initiative in which they were the guinea pigs. They coped well with the hiccups and occasional lack of clarity.

Flexibility

Another lesson learnt was the need to be flexible about the overall project and the individual evaluations. One illustration of this was the timetable for evaluations discussed above. Another was the level and timing of support. The 'implicit' feel of the overall project enabled a great deal of flexibility.

Establishing reasonable autonomy

A third lesson learnt was that of the difficulties of establishing 'reasonable autonomy' to undertake valued evaluation work. The ENG intended from an early point that the evaluators would be given autonomy within quite wide boundaries. In this the project manager had to tread a fine line between support and directing the evaluations. The evaluators felt this had been useful to guide them, but still had the latitude to define their own work. Only one felt the manager's own evaluation agenda had influenced his or her project, but as it had encouraged the evaluator to be more professional, this was conceded as not a bad thing.

It was sometimes harder for the evaluators themselves, and some of the managers and staff of the project being evaluated, to see the need for reasonable autonomy. Approval to interview managers, staff and clients varied across projects. The control of managers over databases of clients was variously exercised. All managers asked to see the questionnaires before they were used: some suggested changes, all of which the evaluators found useful. It is not clear if this was their usual response to evaluators or was a facet of their being community evaluators.

Implicitly good – good for whom?

We will now consider in more depth the underpinning assumptions behind the general idea that the project was a good thing to do. We shall discuss these in turn.

Local, long-term unemployed people as recruits

People were recruited, but their profiles did not match the ENG's conceptualisation of 'long-term' unemployed. It is not clear to what extent interest in such work still exists among the long-term unemployed, or whether this was a one-off recruitment. This has implications for a future recruitment strategy of a similar project.

It may be that in a future recruitment the idea of 'community working', something the evaluators said appealed to them, should be emphasised through community groups. Non-academic skills, such as listening, may also need to be stressed.

Providing recruits with support

They were able to undertake the work, but it took more resources to achieve this than was originally envisaged, notably in terms of the direct support of the line manager. It may be that less qualified people would have required more direct support. Largely this lack of foresight was a result of the project's initially being given an emphasis and lead from a 'job creation scheme' point of view.

Employing people on the minimum wage

That this was fair is an assumption that has still not been properly debated in the ENG. The initial debate halted at being a practical means, and a right one, to provide the community evaluators with a step back into work.

However, the evaluators consistently raised the issue of remuneration. Their concerns were twofold. First, with the responsibility they had – of interviewing a range of people, potentially working in the evening, going into people's homes and writing a report – why were they being paid the same as those on the domestic cleaner training course? Second, if they were being paid so little, their work surely could not be valued or taken seriously by those who commissioned it? This variously influenced their self-confidence, self-image and ability to come to terms with their 'reasonable autonomy'.

The work that they have produced, however, is largely of a high, professional standard. Putting aside any general concerns over the minimum wage and fairness, it does seem to be rather small remuneration for evaluation work, especially given the fees consultants can command. A greater emphasis on 'evaluation' at the beginning might have raised more concern, debate and even resolution over this.

Worthwhile, respect-worthy evaluation

The evaluators have produced reports that are, to varying degrees, being taken note of in planning future developments in Wolverhampton. This is despite the fact that they do not have an already accepted 'professional' or 'academic' letterhead for their work. Concerted efforts have been made to represent their work at influential meetings and to develop a local dissemination strategy which offers comments and the reports to senior members of the organisations concerned.

Longer-term employment opportunities

Two of the evaluators have already secured career jobs. One left the project after a couple of months to take up a two-year contract as a research assistant at the University of Wolverhampton. Having a master's degree and a desire to do this kind of work were the main factors in helping her to obtain the post, but she believed being involved in the project had increased her confidence and had given her the practical experience she had hitherto been lacking. Another was offered the position of learning mentor in a local secondary school. She felt applying for the job from an 'in employment' status had helped her in this achievement. She also felt that she had acquired transferable skills through the work and had been involved in something that created a good impression of her capability, rather than having a lower status job.

Everyone commented that undertaking the work had helped them to get into a routine of work and boosted their confidence. They felt that this would help them to find longer-term employment.

Perhaps one of the most significant successes in terms of continuing to develop the theme of community evaluation has been the contract extension for four months, with higher pay, for three of the evaluators. Current ad hoc interest in using the evaluators for individual projects may build in momentum to a systematic approach towards local evaluation consultants.

A cheaper way of undertaking evaluation?

Running the project was not cheap. The cocktail of funding meant that the direct cost to the HAZ was small, and thus appeared cheap. However, if the trained evaluators are lost to the organisation and the process has to begin again from scratch, then a large part of the investment, especially of time, is lost.

Community evaluators and HAZ values

The community evaluators have enormously helped the ENG to cover its wide remit of evaluating the HAZ. They have directly reported evaluations of projects, and their socioeconomic data helps to provide a wider perspective on the impact of the HAZ. It is not clear, however, whether or not the evaluators have helped the ENG to develop an overall evaluation culture for the HAZ. Interest in evaluation may have been sparked more by developments regarding budget allocation after the initial HAZ period.

Community evaluators as opposed to external evaluators

It is untested as to whether community evaluators have added something to the evaluation that external evaluators would have missed. It is not clear that an extra 'community' perspective has been added to evaluation through this project.

Community evaluators could act as 'honest brokers' between communities and organisational development

Again, this is a largely untested assumption. A longer period is required to see the impact of the community evaluators' work. It seems clear, though, that their work is likely to have more impact (on community involvement and actual services) if the initiative is seen as a learning step for a programme of community evaluation, rather than as a one-off or ad hoc employment project.

A first step in a wider programme of community engagement and capacity building

This is yet another assumption that requires a longer perspective than we are able to provide right now. The warm feeling of the project being a 'good' initiative is still there and, indeed, has spread beyond the initial project team. This and other models of community evaluation are now being used across Wolverhampton. These efforts are, however, a little disjointed and the overall impact is lost.

Some of the resources put into this project have been lost to the HAZ and health and social care in Wolverhampton. As we have noted, some of the evaluators have moved on to other things. The lack of any longer-term planning to store the investment in the community evaluators for future health and social care evaluation was a failing. This partly arose from the fact that this was a new project for those involved, and from the early 'employment' focus. It is something that we are hoping to address. There is interest in strategically improving the evaluation capacity within health and social care in Wolverhampton. This would include a community-led perspective to draw activity together and capture best practice.

It is probably not the case that the initiative increased overall community capacity to influence and be engaged with health and social care. The short-term nature of the project worked against this. If the project is used as a stepping stone to a more systematic approach to community evaluation it could have a key role to play in community engagement.

Conclusion

The overly implicit genesis of the project has had several consequences for its development. The general feeling that it was a 'good' thing to do helped it to make progress, acquire widespread support and develop a flexible approach. The community evaluators themselves certainly valued much of their loose remit (aside from such issues as a desire for tighter deadlines). This allowed them to find a pace and approach that suited them, and allowed them to discover their own potential.

The fact that the implicit assumptions took most explicit hold in the early phase around an 'employment creation' focus created a legacy that had to be pragmatically dealt with during the course of the project. Most notably, this concerned the lack of planning for the level of direct support given to the evaluators in the course of their work.

Some very positive comments can be made about the project's achievements. Firstly, the timely nature of the initiative: articles are beginning to appear either heralding a government initiative involving local workers or, like the present chapter, outlining a project newly completed.

A second achievement has been a substantial raising of awareness of evaluation in Wolverhampton, both in terms of what it can achieve and how it can be done, among the project managers and workstream leads. Evaluation, for many managers, is a new aspect they are being encouraged to include in their project design, and they are keen to think about 'user perception' or 'problem areas' as a focus of the evaluation. The socioeconomic profiling of HAZ service users has added to discussions of what 'reducing inequalities' means in our work. Managers also feel able to engage with the project's 'localness', rather than with the usual university or consultant.

Most notable has been the acknowledgement of the initiative by the HAZ Review Group. Different routes to mainstreaming the work are being discussed, and an initial proposal of an Evaluation Unit has been presented to the Health and Social Care Board to consider. We would like to continue the formative evaluation work and extend the Unit's remit to focus on community involvement in R&D, and to undertake staff development and facilitation to enable widespread use of evaluation in Wolverhampton.

Judging by the high response rates from the evaluators' postal surveys (over 60% for a couple of the larger projects), the public are willing to be surveyed as a means to improve service delivery in the city.

CHAPTER 6

Wakefield and District Health Action Zone: partnerships and learning

Lee Adams, Pete Alcock and Graham Brown

Introduction

The Wakefield and District Health Action Zone (HAZ) was established in the second round of HAZs in 1999. It was based on a joint submission from the then health authority and local authority, and was developed to address some of the serious problems of poor public health known to be present in the district. The district of Wakefield, a former coal mining and industrial area with high levels of chronic heart disease, cancer and a range of other industrial health problems, has a population of some 318,000.

The health authority and local authority had coterminous boundaries, and the HAZ was based on these. This provided a clear political and organisational base for partnership development and joint working, an advantage not shared by many other HAZs. However, in common with other HAZs (Maddock, 2000; Unwin and Westland, 2000), Wakefield and District HAZ had at its core a desire to improve and develop partnership modes of working – focusing these across five core objectives outlined in the initial bid for funding:

- build community participation and capacity
- promote positive health and prevent disease
- tackle the root causes of ill health
- develop integrated health and social care services
- create a Wakefield District HAZ culture and infrastructure (Wakefield HAZ, 1999).

A multi-agency team comprising elements of health authority, local authority and NHS Community Trust staff resources manages the programme. Collectively, this staff team is known as Wakefield Action for Health. The HAZ programme is likewise managed by a multi-agency HAZ Coordinating Group.

Despite the advantage of coterminous boundaries, however, the district has suffered from a long tradition of a lack of true partnership working, and some traditional distrust between statutory agencies, notably the local authority and the health authority and local health trusts. The HAZ commitment to partnership working thus began its development in a cold climate, where much effort had to be put into networking between agencies, and building trust and confidence in co-working (HDA, 2001).

Many partnership bodies have come into being in recent years in the district, though mainly for the purposes of administering the funding regimes of the Single Regeneration Budget (SRB) and various EU programmes (Taylor, 1997; Gregory, 1998). The question here, though, is one of authentic district-wide partnership working, which it is clear has not had a long history in the district. A report published by the Charities Information Bureau (1999) pointed out, in commenting on the state of the voluntary and community sectors, that it was 'underdeveloped', and that there was a 'relative lack of resources at the district-wide level' (p. 2) for the sectors. The voluntary and community sectors are of course just one part of the wider jigsaw of the partnership concept, although they are fundamentally important to the development of genuine partnership working. It is clear from the CIB report that the poorly developed voluntary and community sector is due to what might almost be described as a 'tradition' or culture of a rather wider paternalistic approach to the communities of the district. Adams et al. (2001) reinforce this view, based on the idea of the previously dominant industry of coal mining and associated infrastructures providing much of the social and welfare activities that were required by the communities. Importantly, this model of operation was often carried through into the local authority elected-member body, with many of the local councillors employed in coal mining or at least very closely linked to it.

The point is that ultimately the culture of Wakefield district was one of reliance on a single industry and its linked suppliers, one of anecdotally understood low levels of trust of the voluntary and community sector, one of conventional models of public service delivery and one of low levels of innovative practice. Where change was evident, it was usually a product of national policy requirements or other external demands, quite often linked to securing access to funds. At the heart of the issue, however, were the relationships between those existing people and organisations that currently hold power and those who are seeking to challenge this power, and to share it – supported now by key elements of national government policy.

It was thus into a largely sceptical context that the HAZ was launched in 1999. Prior to this time, though, at the national level, the government had made it clear that it saw new models of public service more favourably and was developing more inclusive approaches (Adams and Brown, 2001; SEU, 2001). Strong evidence of this was seen with the publication of the white papers *Modern local government: in touch with the people* (issued by the Department of the Environment, Transport and the Regions, 1998) and *Modernising government* (issued by the Cabinet Office, 1999). The Social Exclusion Unit was also giving at this time clear signs of its forthcoming views on public services, and local government and health services in particular, through its work on a number of issues and the commitment of the government to continue to support the work of the Unit by broadening the brief the Unit held (SEU, 1999).

It was therefore not an entirely negative picture, despite the local context, within which the HAZ was to operate. Work commenced quickly, leading to the adoption of the HAZ Plan (Wakefield HAZ, 1999), the core elements of which were restated and reaffirmed at a meeting of the HAZ Coordinating Group in October 2001.

At the inception of the HAZ the key features of the evaluation processes to be employed were established. Several key features were felt to be desirable in the evaluation regime, as follows:

- a collaborative approach, with evaluators working closely with the HAZ partners and projects
- the creation of local expertise in evaluation, for reasons of sustainability
- evaluation that is integrated within the HAZ programme.
- an evaluation process that assists with indicator and target development at all levels of the HAZ programme
- the employment of theories of change and realistic evaluation approaches
- a programme-wide strategic process, with in-depth specific case studies.
- a process with a strong academic basis to counteract the problem of having no local higher academic institution, which might otherwise have been involved.

The evaluation work was ultimately placed, after a competitive tendering process, within a collaborative research team comprising members of the Social Policy and Social Work team at Birmingham University and the Federation of Community Work Training Groups' Collective.

The evaluation research methodology is based upon realistic evaluation principles and a 'theories of change' approach. This meant that early on in the evaluation process, at all levels within the HAZ, work was done with participants to identify objectives, indications and milestones. This work was then supplemented by documentary analysis, interviews, questionnaires and workshops at both the strategic level and the project level. However, there is also a commitment to supporting the development of self-evaluation skills and techniques among all HAZ project activities, and as part of this a tailored evaluation handbook was produced for use within the district.

It quickly became clear during the evaluation process that securing improved partnership working was a major priority across all dimensions of HAZ work, and that achievements here would be one of the major learning points for Wakefield. Several other concepts and issues were also closely linked to this central matter of partnership. These included whole systems approaches, the development of social capital, organisational development and community development/involvement. It is difficult to get to the central issue of partnership development without coming across one or more of these related concerns, as in Wakefield all have proved to be inextricably linked. The reasons for this are many. The low level of partnership working, it could be said, is really a reflection of low levels of other types of work and activity, such as community or organisational development, or a lack of embracing social capital as a positive concept, for example.

It is therefore worth discussing these other issues and concepts, and attempting to describe them in terms of learning and development.

Social capital

The HAZ commissioned a report on the theoretical debates and empirical research on social capital from the evaluation team (Alcock and Mason, 2001). This posed the central question, 'Should we invest in social capital?'. It described the concept as linked to social exclusion and inclusive of informal contacts, such as friends and family, social networks of colleagues and acquaintances, associations, learning clubs and other groups and membership of organisations such as formal bodies. Activity at all of these levels is important for the promotion and development of social capital, and the HAZ, and other local agents, have a key role to play in this (Green et al., 2000).

It is clear that Wakefield suffers low levels of social capital and that the approach taken by the HAZ to tackle this has been at two primary levels. The first is at the project level whereby projects have been established with social capital outputs, such as a proposal to establish a volunteer bureau, for example. The second level is that which is woven within all of the work of the HAZ, through the employment of social capital approaches in working with partners (McCabe et al., 2001).

This approach has meant that the concept of high levels of social capital has been seen from the outset as a target within the work of the Action for Health team, linked to community and organisational development approaches, as evidenced by the 2001 evaluation report (Alcock, 2001).

Organisational development

As a result of the broader policy changes initiated within its modernisation pro-gramme, the government has promoted organisational change across the field of public service (Carley et al., 2000a,b; SEU, 2001). At a local level within Wakefield the impact of such changes has meant that the formal organisational development work of the HAZ has been submerged in a sea of wider changes. However, the mode of operation of the HAZ has brought about positive devel-opments in itself, as well as allowing the HAZ to place itself at the heart of the changes as they are developed locally.

This has meant that while the district had relatively low levels of commitment to and experience of partnership planning and collaborative working, the HAZ has succeeded in playing a key catalytic role in shifting policies and practice – a point identified in the most recent annual report of the evaluation team (Alcock, 2001).

The five objectives of the HAZ described above have proved durable and an extremely useful touchstone throughout the life of the HAZ. They have remained the organisational driving force for all activity, and as such have also provided much needed stability in extremely turbulent times.

Nevertheless, the desire to engage in more formal organisational development work, such as the production of an organisational development strategy, has not been realised, mainly because of external forces. The positive lesson, though, is that much can be achieved through leading by example, in policies and everyday practice. The fact is if key organisational principles, formal as well as informal, such as those described by the HAZ objectives, are established and owned by partners, then the organisational development work which can be carried through becomes much easier to achieve, even in the absence of formal organi-sational development strategies.

Community development and involvement

As with organisational development, community development work is funda-mental to the work of the Wakefield HAZ. It is central to the interpretation of the social model of health, which is at the heart of the Wakefield HAZ approach, as articulated in the original HAZ Plan (Wakefield HAZ, 1999).

Wakefield HAZ, as part of the building of social capital, for they are surely two sides of the same coin, has promoted community development work at two main levels. The project level has seen much work at the locality and commu-nity level, targeted at deprived communities of interest and geographic location (Webster, 2000; Smithies, 2001). location. The strategic level has meant that community development approaches are employed in all interactions with peo-ple and communities. This has meant in practice that the promotion of health is seen as dependent to a large extent upon the social and economic health of communities (Wakefield MDC, 2001). High levels of social capital are a positive indicator of a healthy community, for example, and they remind us that we should be concerned not just with the health of the individuals that make up the community, important though that is, but with the health of the collective community itself.

The aim of the community development work is placed within this wider context. In Wakefield, however, the levels of community development activity were extremely low when compared to a number of other HAZ areas. The HAZ is still the only public sector initiative promoting and practising community development work in the district to any significant degree. The HAZ has sought to lead the implementation of community involvement both in practical and policy terms, and to adopt an inclusive approach here. It has commissioned the production of a community involvement strategy for the district (Webster, 2001), but this is still to be adopted by all local agencies.

In practical terms the initial reluctance of the major public sector agencies to get involved in community development work, and their wish only to countenance community involvement at the most cursory level, has presented difficulties. The national pressure to engage with communities, coupled with employment of community development approaches, seems not to have penetrated to the levels required for action to flow. The HAZ community development work has thus remained isolated, and to some extent marginalised. This is bound to impact upon the central question of partnership development, because the capacity of the community and voluntary sectors to get involved at the levels envisaged by the government may well not be present.

On the positive side, the HAZ programme has released much energy in the voluntary and community sectors. The HAZ report (Webster, 2001) provides a blueprint for future work. The continuing HAZ commitment to community development work is having effects in the localities and within the communities benefiting from the work. Certainly for Wakefield HAZ such work has proved invaluable in demonstrating commitment to the promotion of the social model of health, but just as importantly the commitment to different models of engaging with communities has been met in largely positive ways. Some of the comments from an evaluation event held in March 2001 help sum up achievements that have been made here:

- 'Community involvement is a lot higher up the agenda because of the HAZ'
- 'Increased community participation – increased partnership working'
- 'Introduced new culture and approaches' (Wilde et al., 2001, 4).

Whole systems approaches see the organisational world as a set of interdependent, complex factors. That is to say, no organisation can operate in isolation from its environment, including clients, governments, other organisations and even employees (Wilkinson, 1997; Wilkinson and Applebee, 1999).

This is important because it helps us to see the operation of a HAZ programme as just one factor within the complex scene of different organisations and pressures. In practical terms it means that 'we are all in this together' and that actions that, for example, the local authority takes are bound to have an impact on other organisations and on service users. This approach to seeing the linkages between actions in one field and subsequent impact in another goes to the heart of the government approach in the development of community strategies. It has given rise to the often-heard call to 'join things up'.

The general approach, then, is to avoid seeing policies and actions in isolation and to try to establish a clear set of goals for all. The HAZ programme and the Action for Health team are at the centre of this approach, which has now come to encompass the developing local strategic partnership (LSP).

This positive placement of the HAZ has been achieved through a combination of techniques, encompassing the espousal of the social model of health (itself a systemic approach), through to playing a leading role in developing 'professional' multi-agency bodies, such as a local Area-Based Initiatives Group, the Multi-Agency Information Group and the work to develop community involvement.

Partnership working

At the core of all of this work are the concept and practice of partnership working. The national pressures in this area have proved useful, although they have on occasions been counterbalanced by nationally instigated organisational disruption.

In organisational theory terms, partnerships are increasingly seen as the modern response to difficult challenges. In the private sector this can mean that the cost of the development of a microchip can be shared across a partnership, for example (Daft, 1995). Similarly, the public service sector can meet significant challenges in its use of partnerships.

Another dimension of partnership is ownership. If partners are involved in making a collaborative decision then they are more likely to carry through or 'own' the action flowing from that decision (Gregory, 1998; Carley et al., 2000b). Within Wakefield the HAZ is recognised to be a key element in the new and improving culture of collaboration that now exists in the area. It has achieved this through clear objectives that are widely shared by partner agencies – and by the practical efforts of innovative co-working within funded projects.

The development of partnerships and of partnership styles of working has thus been a central plank of the work of Wakefield HAZ. The evaluation process has found much to praise in the work that has been undertaken, but has also found difficulties.

On the positive side, an increased commitment to partnership working is now seen and the HAZ itself is seen as a good example of a partnership approach. Partnership planning is more widely embraced at a strategic level, and partnership working has developed significantly over the first two years of the HAZ, in particular across the major public sector agencies (Wakefield MDC, 2001). Most importantly of all the HAZ has succeeded in acting as a catalyst for partnership working on regeneration, with the Action for Health team being instrumental in the promotion of a cultural shift within the local area.

Some of the problems still to be addressed, however, include the procedural impact of performance management on partners and the Action for Health team, the difficulty of securing commitment to real partnership activity from some mainstream services providers, and the slow progress encountered in some areas in securing financial commitments to mainstream HAZ-funded projects. More generally the adverse financial situation experienced by the HAZ and the uncertainty over future planning have made long-term partnership planning more difficult to develop and sustain.

Despite these difficulties, however, it is clear that the HAZ had a positive effect on partnership development. The existence of the HAZ, in its adaptation of key partnership principles and its promotion of such principles to other bodies, has been almost universally positive. The coincidence of government action on community strategies, LSPs and on 'joining things up' has helped locally. However, given the low levels of capacity to exploit such initiatives that existed prior to the implementation of the HAZ, it is doubtful that much progress would have been made without the HAZ.

Conclusions

Partnership working is clearly important and the HAZ, both in its own field and beyond, has been able, through policy and practice, to promote and develop such ways of working. Partnership working is also at the heart of the much government activity, and Wakefield HAZ has been able to exploit this external pressure successfully.

It is clear that partnership working in itself is impossible to separate from the linked issues of social capital, community development, organisational development and whole systems thinking. All of these elements have to be in place at least to some degree to enable genuine partnership working to develop.

Partnership working is not easy and it certainly is not a quick fix, as evidenced through the work of Wakefield HAZ and its evaluation processes. However, a positive start has been made which requires more time to develop and implement. The development of trust between partners is one of the main developmental factors. This itself, though, is dependent upon the clarification of power relationships. Genuine partnerships need an understanding that trust is required, but that power relationships will be challenged. This is a process, and a challenge, which has been begun in Wakefield, but which still has some way to go.

References

Adams, L. and Brown, G. (2001) 'Healthy communities and the impact of government modernisation policy: a paper for the Nuffield Institute for Health' [unpublished].

Adams, L., Brown, G., Duggan, M. and Pollock, C. (2001) *Inequalities in health: causes and solutions*, Wakefield: Wakefield HAZ.

Alcock, P. (2001) *Summary evaluation report, 2000/01*, Wakefield: Wakefield HAZ.

Alcock, P. and Mason, P. (2001) *Should we invest in social capital?*, Wakefield: Wakefield HAZ.

Carley, M., Campbell, M., Kearns, A., Wood, M. and Young, R. (2000a) *Regeneration in the 21st century: policies into practice*, Bristol: Policy Press.

Carley, M., Chapman, M., Hastings, A., Kirk, K. and Young, R. (2000b) *Urban regeneration through partnership*, Bristol: Policy Press.

Charities Information Bureau (1999) *Social inclusion and regeneration*, Wakefield: CIB.

Daft, R. (1995) *Organisation theory and design*, St Paul, Minnesota: West.

Green, G., Grimley, M., Suokas, A., Prescott, M., Jowitt, T. and Linacre, R. (2000) *Social capital, health and economy in South Yorkshire coalfield communities*, Sheffield: Sheffield Hallam University.

Gregory, S. (1998) *Transforming local services: partnership in action*, York: YPS.

HDA (2001) *Ideas and proposals for promoting healthy communities*, London: HDA.

Maddock, S. (2000) 'Managing the development of partnerships in Health Action Zones', *International Journal of Health Care Quality Assurance*, 13/2 (2000), 65–73.

McCabe, A., Wilde, P. and Wilson, M. (2001) *Project case studies evaluation report, 2000–01*, Wakefield: Wakefield HAZ.

SEU (1999) *Review of the Social Exclusion Unit*, London: SEU.

SEU (2001) *A new commitment to neighbourhood renewal: national strategy action plan*, London: SEU.

Smithies J. (2001) *Community development in Wakefield*, Wakefield: Wakefield Community Development Steering Group.

Taylor, M. (1997) *The best of both worlds: the voluntary sector and local government*, York: YPS.

Unwin, J. and Westland, P. (2000) *Health Action Zones: the engagement of the voluntary sector*, London: The Baring Foundation.

Wakefield HAZ (1999) *A healthier life for all*, Wakefield: Wakefield HAZ.

Wakefield MDC (2001) *The Wakefield community strategy 2001*, Wakefield: Wakefield WMDC.

Webster, G. (2000) *Mapping community involvement strategies and mechanisms across Wakefield District*, Wakefield: Wakefield HAZ.

Webster, G. (2001) *Getting people involved*, Wakefield: Wakefield HAZ.

Wilde, P., Wilson, M. and Harris, V. (2001) *End of year evaluation event, 6 March 2001: summary of discussions*, Wakefield: Wakefield HAZ.

Wilkinson, D. (1997) 'Whole system development: rethinking public service management', *International Journal of Public Sector Management*, 10/7, 505–33.

Wilkinson, D. and Applebee, E. (1999) *Implementing holistic government*, Bristol: Policy Press.

CHAPTER 7

A role for Health Action Zones within local strategic partnerships: lessons from the South-West

Joyce Halliday, Sue Richardson and Sheena Asthana

Introduction

In the South-West of England the Health Action Zone (HAZ) concept encompasses two adjacent but highly dissimilar zones. The first covers the tightly bounded city of Plymouth with a population of 255,000, the second the whole of the largely rural and maritime county of Cornwall together with the Isles of Scilly (C&IoS). Here the population approaches some 500,000, but it is 132 kilometres from the north-eastern boundary at Morwenstow to Land's End, while the Isles of Scilly lie a further 45 kilometres to the west.

Amid the continuing uncertainty surrounding both the future of HAZs and the function and form of local strategic partnerships (LSPs), this paper draws on learning from these two contrasting areas, where both HAZs have invested significantly in evaluation, to explore the likely contribution of HAZs to LSPs. Specifically, it examines how these two HAZs are participating in the LSP development process and asks what lessons for LSPs can be drawn from the HAZ experience to date.

Background

The final government guidance on local strategic partnerships was published by the Department of the Environment, Transport and the Regions in March 2001 (DETR, 2001). The aim is to bring together the public, private, voluntary and community sectors to improve the delivery of public services and the quality of life of people at the local level. In this LSPs are critical to implementing the government's National Strategy for Neighbourhood Renewal, a programme to tackle deprivation focused on 88 deprived neighbourhoods, and it is here that the imperative for development and accreditation is the strongest (see DTLR, 2001). But LSPs also have a much wider remit. They are expected to develop across England and play a key strategic role in developing community strategies, in bringing together and looking at ways to rationalise partnership and planning arrangements, and in developing and delivering on local public service agreements (DETR, 2001).

Both the agenda and the current emphasis on accreditation within local authorities eligible for Neighbourhood Renewal Funds suggest an important role for local government. However, the government guidance is emphatic in requiring that LSPs 'actively involve all the key players' (DETR, 2001). The health community in general has thus been urged to recognise the significance of these initiatives and the importance of early engagement. This included an expectation at the outset that health authorities (alongside the wider health community) would help determine how health interests should be represented, ensure the health input to LSPs is properly coordinated, ensure that strategies are developed for delivering national priorities and targets, and ensure that Health Improvement Programmes (HImPs) and PCT plans are aligned with community planning arrangements and neighbourhood renewal strategies (Milburn, 2001).

At the same time the government guidance, together with the NHS Plan, also acknowledged that HAZs should have a valuable contribution to make to the general development of LSPs, and suggested that in the medium term they could be integrated into these partnerships 'to strengthen the links between health, education, employment and other sources of social exclusion' (DoH, 2000). Indeed, it was expected that they would 'be able to contribute resources, including funding, to LSP strategies and projects that impact on the health of people in local communities' (DETR, 2001).

The subsequent move towards strategic health authorities, with its concomitant organisational insecurity and the associated impact on organisational status and managerial capacity, has reduced the ability of health authorities to be proactive in securing the position of health within this critical new arena. Similar tensions may inhibit the degree to which HAZs can influence the process. Their initial funding period is drawing to a close, staff are concerned to mainstream successful projects and demonstrate the achievements of their initiative, and, while the indications for continued government support for the HAZ initiative beyond April 2002 are good, confirmation is not likely before January 2002. There are thus immediate difficulties for any HAZ in attempting to engage meaningfully with an emerging partnership when its own future remains uncertain (both in terms of funding and focus).

This is compounded by the realisation that a HAZ's efficacy (and indeed its continued existence) may be judged in part by its ability to permeate this new political space. In some areas it has been suggested that HAZs are already playing a leading role in LSP development. Certainly, the Department of Health would like to see this role developed further, yet it is recognised that this is 'subject to the local pace of LSP development' and likely to develop faster in some areas than others, a factor which again sits uneasily alongside the continued reticence over the future of the HAZ initiative. In our two case study HAZs, for example, Plymouth has the incentive of Neighbourhood Renewal Funding but this applies to only part of Cornwall, the two western districts of Penwith and Kerrier.

Initial reactions from the HAZs

Both HAZs in the South-West have adopted a proactive stance in the development of local LSPs – initiating meetings with strategic players in their localities, seeking appropriate representation, and supporting the LSP process by variously encouraging debate, breaking down boundaries and resourcing structures. A cynical explanation might be that, with the continued uncertainties over the HAZ initiative itself, LSPs represent a potential lifeline and a possible arena for continuing strategic influence. However, the evidence from C&IoS and Plymouth suggests a more optimistic interpretation, with the HAZ teams perceiving themselves to be a key resource with distinctive experience that can contribute positively to the local strategic agenda.

There is indeed a considerable commonality of concern between the two agendas, and just as LSPs are required to 'build on best practice from successful partnerships', the HAZs have placed a considerable emphasis on evaluation, the need to learn from new initiatives and new ways of working, and the need to disseminate this learning to effect. This chapter draws on the evaluations under way in C&IoS and Plymouth HAZs to offer some lessons for the developing LSPs.

Sustaining the HAZ ethos

Both HAZs have been at least partly responsible for recent changes in the perception of 'health'. They aim to tackle health inequalities, and this encompasses both a greater recognition of the broader determinants of health, including social inclusion and involvement, and a greater acceptance and understanding of the beneficial effect of health, in its broadest sense, on the regeneration of the locality.

An important corollary has been a change in the perceptions that people have of 'health' and of 'health people'. In both Cornwall and the Isles of Scilly and

Plymouth the HAZs are credited with bringing partners together where this had not previously proved possible. Different explanations for this have been posited, including the incentive of additional resources. It is widely believed, though, that the fact that the HAZs have demonstrated that they are different from 'old health' has played no small part in this achievement. Even within the 'traditional enclaves' of the health world, horizons are widening and new ways of seeing health are being incorporated. The HAZs are not only thus crossing sector boundaries, they are also concerned with working across the boundaries within the health sector itself.

The fact that the HAZ is seen as 'doing things differently' thus has the potential for facilitating cooperation and partnership. However, it also carries the potential for polarisation. If the HAZ is perceived as being positive to partnership working by those in non-health sectors, it is possible that those involved with the HAZ will be welcomed while others within 'health' will not. Efforts to embrace a more fluid definition of health will need to be made in all parts of the health world to ensure that aspects or individuals not associated with the HAZ are not isolated. Conversely, there is evidence that 'HAZ champions' are not always satisfied that health representation alone is sufficient to ensure that the HAZ ethos will be sustained.[1]

When it comes to thinking about LSPs, then, careful consideration will need to be given to any representation from the health community, and it should be recognised that, at least for now, HAZ and 'health' are not necessarily synonymous.

Partnership working

The guidance on LSPs emphasises the need to build on existing partnerships while strengthening, deepening and broadening the membership and structure, and considering barriers to involvement. The evaluations of partnership effectiveness in the case study HAZs corroborate the difficulties evidenced in the partnership literature. Partnerships are expensive, the demands are frequently underestimated and the necessary resources, in particular dedicated time, are frequently lacking. Effective partnership requires vision and enthusiasm, commitment at the right level, and trust between partners that can withstand external pressures on individual organisations or groups.

Results from a survey of partnership achievements and constraints conducted with the strategic representatives steering the C&IoS HAZ suggested that con-

---

[1] Interestingly, the Department of Health LSP tour report (DoH, 2001) found similar concerns over the ability of one organisation to represent the local health community, and a strong feeling that representing health and representing the NHS were not the same tasks.

siderable progress had been made in this direction. There is, for example, strong agreement that stakeholders now recognise and accept the need for partnership, and have been able to ensure commitment and ownership. Less progress has been made in terms of developing and maintaining trust or nurturing a partnership culture in individual organisations. Achievements often stop short of the point at which pooled budgets are created, tensions remain where responsibilities are to be ceded or assumed and, under stress, it remains easier to act within the confines of a single agency, where the rules for working are transparent and accessible, than in a multi-agency environment.

Clear leadership and lines of accountability are also vital requisites, as is good communication. Preliminary evidence in the South-West suggests a lack of appreciation of the level of support needed for such information and knowledge management. For example, in Plymouth the HAZ is supported by three administrative officers and a communications manager. This team is responsible for the day-to-day running of the HAZ, as well as providing administrative support for each of the 12 programme boards and communicating with the local press and local partnerships, and with national groups such as HAZnet, individual HAZs, and the HAZ National Evaluation Team. There is thus little capacity left for the management of knowledge within the HAZ itself. However, this is becoming increasingly important as HAZs realise their role as 'learning organisations'. There is, for instance, an increasing amount of knowledge to be shared between programmes as evaluative lessons emerge locally, as well a wealth of relevant national and international evidence-based information. With 64 individual projects across 12 largely autonomous programme boards, and many stakeholders in the wider community, simply locating the people who need a certain piece of information can be a complex task when the systems are not in place to support such activity. Given that LSPs are tasked with a coordination role, this may be an important lesson.

Clarity of purpose is also critical to the effectiveness of partnerships (see e.g. Evans and Killoran, 2000) and this has again been borne out by the local evaluation. Here the changing national agenda, the need to concentrate on tackling health inequalities and on modernising services, the tension between a desire to work in new ways and the need to meet performance targets, the uneasy juxtaposition of community involvement and a time-limited initiative, for instance, have variously dissipated clarity of purpose, but at least there has been a unified focus on improving health. In contrast, LSPs could find themselves pulled not in many directions within a single overarching objective but in many different directions within a stream of interrelated objectives.

Attention needs also to be paid to the *level* of partnership working (Nuffield Institute for Health, 1998): it can be easier for partners to agree to do something (strategic) than to agree how, precisely, to do it (operational). This has been observed in both Plymouth and Cornwall and the Isles of Scilly, in, for example moves towards integrated services. This ability to move from planning to implementation is vital to achieve the real benefits that are being sought from partnership working. As one programme board chair put it, 'People judge by the tangible expression of benefits on the ground, not by mission statements'. The HAZs have sometimes struggled with implementing agreed policy but there is evidence of success. The HAZ partnerships are beginning to be seen locally as partnerships that can deliver.

This is well illustrated in Cornwall where the HAZ project manager, members of the HAZ project team and HAZ champions have secured increasingly influential positions within the economic regeneration arena. Objective One is proving a particularly critical interface. It represents a major source of new money within the county, but is an area where health, despite the presence of the Objective One director on the HAZ Steering Group, has for a long time been marginalised, largely by virtue of technical restrictions on eligible projects. Yet, at the same time, both at the strategic level and at the local level, via the Integrated Area Plan (IAP) structures, Objective One is emerging as a key agent in the LSP equation.

Significantly, the HAZ project manager has now not only been asked to join the Community Futures Taskforce (the aim of which is to encourage and support projects which address issues of social inclusion and community regeneration to apply for Objective One funding) but also to play a potentially pivotal role in facilitating proposals to the fund. This is testament not only to the foresight and persistence on the part of the HAZ in recognising the need to gain representation on this forum, but also to the recognition in regeneration circles that the HAZ can be an effective ally in a partnership that works. Here the combination of its established county-wide framework and local delivery mechanisms (using the HAZ community health development model) is seen as capable of assisting Objective One in delivering earmarked funds for the most deprived wards in Cornwall.

Community involvement

Another key partnership challenge faced by the HAZs, and currently facing emerging LSPs, is the need to involve small organisations, community groups and the wider public in a meaningful way. This means that community and user involvement is increasingly seen as a necessary foundation for both project and policy development, or, in the LSP context, for the strategic and local alike, rather than as a difficult and externally imposed challenge.

The members of the LSP will firstly need to agree the value of involving communities, and then make available the mechanisms and structures to facilitate this in practice. This again includes resources, information and trust, together with the skills to work with and empower local people. It also includes the recognition that all stakeholders need not necessarily be involved in the same way. There is a concern that voluntary and community involvement is too often dictated by the need 'to achieve targets for the agency concerned', rather than reflecting the needs of the people concerned or actually creating more effective agency working.

At the programme and project level, the two HAZs have involved a very wide range of bodies. The Healthy Living Initiatives Programme within C&IoS HAZ, for example, is informed by a county-wide network of healthy living forums, and supports an active and fast-growing healthy living network where members can shape and access training, and pool resources and experience. The community health development projects it sponsors, together with the support given to the Healthy Living Centre process, actively embrace a wider definition of health and wellbeing, and challenge the ways in which agencies have traditionally divided up the concerns of the community. Nevertheless, the involvement of a cross-spectrum of individuals has been harder to achieve. Again evidence suggests this is an acknowledged challenge and an area where the HAZs are now taking a proactive stance. In North Cornwall, for instance, the Healthy Living Forum has drawn on a HAZ pilot project to explore statutory responses to a dramatic rep-resentation of the problems facing young people as they attempt to make informed health choices, and also used it, via a newsletter, as a springboard to discussing opportunities for young people locally and a mechanism for drawing a wider spectrum of people into the forum itself.

In Plymouth the LSP will undoubtedly find lessons to be learnt from the HAZ when it comes to community involvement. This is not to say that the HAZ provides a perfect model of how to engage with the local community, but it is learning – from its mistakes as well as from its achievements. From the out-set the HAZ voiced a desire for strong involvement from the community and voluntary sector. Indeed, one of the twelve programme boards is concerned specifically with community and voluntary sector development, the idea being that this programme could develop the capacity for involvement in the other eleven programmes. In addition it was decided that there should be a policy of representation from the voluntary and community sector to each of the other eleven programme boards. For a variety of reasons, voluntary sector involvement has been stronger than community involvement in the HAZ, and there are still many communities in Plymouth (both geographical and interest communities) that do not feel engaged with the HAZ. This imbalance has now been recognised within the HAZ, and greater efforts are being made to include communities across the city. Effective use of existing mechanisms, such as the Plymouth

Community Partnership, is hoped to be one way of improving the 'reach' into the community.

The guidance for local strategic partnerships provides a number of expectations about community involvement in LSPs, but precisely how this will be achieved is left to the partnerships themselves. The lessons from the HAZs suggest that LSPs should not use the existence of the Community Empowerment Fund as a substitute for sound processes and structures for community involvement. The funding will assist communities to play a more active role, but without explicit mechanisms in place to facilitate communication, and foster both development and involvement, this will not happen effectively.

Creating and valuing resources

The HAZ has shown by example that, given a nurturing environment, it is possible for partnerships to create vital resources (most importantly, human) and that these need to be valued and further cultivated. In the examples above, HAZ funding is seen not only as helping pump-prime community involvement but also enabling HAZ ways of working to be mainstreamed across partner organisations, so offering support for the process of organisational change.

Individual change can also be a significant resource for the development of future partnerships. At one level perhaps this would encompass the so-called 'HAZ champions' – individuals who now carry aspects of the HAZ way of working into their daily practices. As personnel have moved, this resource has increasingly spread beyond the HAZ project teams, the HAZ project leads, and programme boards. One manager in Plymouth HAZ, when interviewed about his move to a new partnership, for example, said that he wanted to take the HAZ way of doing things with him. He characterised this as 'inclusiveness, openness and transparency'. Similarly, in Cornwall, as staff move from HAZ-affiliated jobs into other local organisations there is a strong feeling that they will 'not retreat into camps' but will continue to promote openness, network, and learn from mistakes as well as successes, 'approaches that have brought fruit here'.

A specific example is provided by the Restormel Regeneration Partnership, formally established in December 2000 to provide a 'holistic approach' to regeneration initiatives within the borough of Restormel. With the inception of the Objective One Integrated Area Plan process, the board agreed that it should take on the responsibility of an accountable body under the IAP umbrella, and became a company limited by guarantee in order to fulfil that function.

Interestingly, contrary to many of the other IAP partnerships, the Restormel partnership has a very strong emphasis on community development rather than an exclusive focus on economic regeneration. One contributory factor is the influence of the vice-chair, who is a primary care group (PCG) chief executive, a member of the HAZ Steering Group and a confirmed HAZ champion. He has both carried the HAZ ethos into the partnership as an individual, and has helped institutionalise it by ensuring the associated values were recognised in the appointment of a project officer with not only wide health and social care interests but previous experience of working in an area with HAZ and Objective One status.

Acknowledging context

Finally, it is not possible to discuss the possible place of health within LSPs without consideration of the local context. One of the most significant factors to have come from a contextual analysis in the South-West is that of coterminosity. This is not a new finding (Exworthy and Peckham, 1999) but its importance may so far have been underestimated. The differences between the two case study HAZs in this respect are stark and will be no less important for LSPs than for the HAZs.

Plymouth can consider itself fortunate in that the HAZ boundaries are coterminous with many others. The HAZ is coterminous with the unitary authority, the PCT, the Pathfinder Plymouth 2020 Partnership (likely to become the LSP) and many other area-based initiatives. In contrast, in Cornwall and the Isles of Scilly the HAZ covers five primary care trusts or groups, works with one county council, six district councils and one unitary authority. The reorganisation of the health authorities is likely to bring even greater difficulties for Cornwall in this respect (with the HAZ losing coterminosity with arguably its most strategic partner, the health authority). It means that it is even more difficult to predict the most appropriate placing for the HAZ and how health should fit within the LSPs.

The general expectation within Cornwall, for instance, has been that there will be a county-wide partnership and a number of more locally based partnerships (perhaps six in total) for a population of about 500,000, with the HAZ possibly serving as a health taskforce to the county-wide partnership. The first challenge for this rural HAZ (and indeed for many other partnerships and organisations within the county) is thus determining how to negotiate the plethora of new partnerships within the context of both limited resources and geographically dispersed and distant loci. The second challenge is how to ensure that health in its widest dimension, in its HAZ livery so to speak, is effectively represented, suggesting that the mainstreaming of the wider HAZ 'way of working' still has some way to go within the health community itself. Again, the structure of the HAZ appears to be a potentially significant determinant in shaping this debate, as do the importance of personality and the movement of personnel between the HAZ project team and the developing primary care organisations.

In Plymouth, in contrast, the new city-wide PCT is consolidating its own organisational shape and considering its relationship with both the HAZ and the emerging LSP, the Plymouth 2020 Partnership (P2020P). This partnership is already benefiting from the support of the HAZ in a number of ways. The HAZ has, for instance, invested much effort through its Voluntary and Community Sector Development Programme Board to improve the involvement of both the voluntary and community sectors in health and social care policy-making and service delivery in Plymouth, and this programme board is now a foundation group for the P2020P and is likely to play a key role in developing the community strategy for the LSP. Likewise, the HAZ Social Exclusion Programme Board has re-formed to create another P2020P foundation group, the Social Inclusion Partnership for Plymouth.

The problems faced by largely non-coterminous partnerships are so greatly amplified in comparison with the largely coterminous partnerships that we would argue strongly that additional resources should be provided specifically where there is a significant level of non-coterminosity.

Conclusion

It is clear that for Plymouth and Cornwall and the Isles of Scilly, the HAZ will be important in the development and continued life of their local strategic partnerships. How closely the two initiatives will be interwoven has yet to be decided, but the HAZs are proving significant in a number of ways. They have significant learning to impart, they can bring direct influence to bear on the shaping of the LSPs, and they have a potentially critical role to play in representing the wide health agenda and an ability to influence the culture of partnership working that the LSPs adopt. They may also have a symbolic significance, for a premature end could be perceived both as a reflection of a lack of government commitment to local partnerships, with consequent implications for the effectiveness of partnership working, and as a signal of the relative importance attached to reducing health inequalities, as opposed to improving service delivery. In either instance it might be increasingly difficult for LSPs to secure the genuine partnership commitment they will need to be effective.

References

DETR (2001) *Local strategic partnerships: government guidance*, London: Department of the Environment, Transport and the Regions.
DoH (2000) *The NHS Plan*, London: Stationery Office.

DoH (2001) 'LSP tour report: internal (unpublished) paper giving feedback from the meetings'.

DTLR (2001b) *Accreditation guidance for local strategic partnerships*, October, London: Department of the Environment, Transport and the Regions.

Evans, D. and Killoran, A. (2000) 'Tackling health inequalities through partnership working: learning from a realistic evaluation', *Critical Public Health*, 10/2, 125–40.

Exworthy, M. and Peckham, S. (1999) 'Collaboration between health and social care: coterminosity in the "New NHS"', *Health and Social Care in the Community*, 7/3, 225–32.

Milburn, A. (2001) 'Local strategic partnerships: government guidance', 4 April [letter; http://www.haznet.org.uk/resources/book_lsp-let.doc]

Nuffield Institute for Health, Community Care Division (1998) 'Inter-agency collaboration: final report', Update, 6, 1–6.

Section 2

Generating learning

Mhairi Mackenzie, Louise Lawson and Jane Mackinnon

From their inception Health Action Zones were expected to be learning organisations. HAZs are therefore required not only to effect change within their local communities but, in addition, to promote local and national understanding of how and why change has occurred.

The complexity of initiatives such as HAZs, however, raises a set of challenges for evaluators. In this foreword we:

- look at the features of HAZs that make them resistant to traditional evaluation approaches
- summarise the approach that has been adopted by the national evaluation team
- consider the implications of this approach for local evaluation
- briefly outline the issues raised by the contributing chapters.

Evaluation challenges

HAZs were established with the aim of reducing health inequalities through the modernisation of services and the building of local capacity for collaboration. In many ways, therefore, they resemble comprehensive community initiatives (CCIs) as described by Connell and Kubisch (1998). The aims of CCIs are: to promote positive changes at the individual, family and community level; to develop a variety of mechanisms to improve social, economic and physical circumstances, services and conditions in disadvantaged communities; and to place a strong emphasis on community building and neighbourhood empowerment.

These characteristics pose a number of challenges for evaluation that can be summarised as follows:

- Initiatives such as HAZs have multiple and broad goals, and are therefore not well suited to evaluation methods that rely on a small number of key outcomes.

- HAZs are highly complex learning enterprises with multiple strands of activity operating at many different levels, from the small project to the most strategic cross-agency, area-based approaches.

- Objectives are defined and strategies are chosen to achieve goals that often change over time. For example, interventions which aim to be locally driven require to respond to community needs, and these are not necessarily defined at the outset; likewise, HAZs frequently find themselves in the position of responding to changing policy requirements at a national level, and this can militate against an entirely stable strategic approach.

- Many activities and intended outcomes are difficult to measure, since units of action are complex, open systems in which it is virtually impossible to control all the variables that may influence the conduct and outcome of evaluation.

- The saturation of a given community with a particular intervention limits further the potential for traditional experimental designs, since the option of randomising individuals to treatment and control is not a viable one. In addition, the possibility of identifying control areas is severely curtailed where an initiative such as a HAZ is implemented on a large scale, and where processes which have been introduced within HAZs are rolled out nationwide before any formal evaluation has taken place.

- Improving health outcomes that are socially determined takes longer than the life span of an initiative and its evaluation.

If complex initiatives are to generate useful learning then there is a demonstrable need to look beyond traditional approaches to evaluation. Increasingly, within the US, Australia, Canada and the UK, theory-based approaches to evaluation are viewed as a potentially useful means of evaluating processes and outcomes in community-based programmes that were not adequately addressed by existing approaches.

National HAZ evaluation: 'theories of change'

One approach that follows the logic of theory-based evaluation and that has informed the work of the national evaluation of HAZs is the 'theories of change' approach developed by the Aspen Institute from its evaluation of comprehensive community interventions in the US.

This theory of change approach is defined as 'a systematic and cumulative study of the links between activities, outcomes and contexts of the initiative' (Connell and Kubisch, 1998). The approach aims to clarify the overall vision or theory of change of the initiative, meaning the long-term outcomes and the strategies that are intended to produce them. In generating this theory, steps are taken to link the original problem or context in which the programme began with the activities planned to address the problem, and the medium and longer-term outcomes intended.

This framework has much in common with the development in the UK of 'realistic evaluation', the second theoretical framework upon which the national HAZ evaluation has drawn. Realistic evaluation can be summarised as an approach that links the context of an initiative with the mechanism chosen to achieve change and the outcomes that emerge over time. A successful evaluation will identify context–mechanism–outcome (CMO) configurations and distinguish between those that do and do not work, in order to refine policy development in the future.

Figure 1 illustrates the general approach that we are taking and encouraging within HAZs themselves. The starting point is for the initiative at an overall programme, workstream and individual project level to reflect on the key aspects of the context within which it is operating. The next stage is to specify a rationale for intervening in relation to priority issues (for example, in response to a local needs assessment). This rationale should then translate into clearly defined change mechanisms, each with specified targets that should form part of a logical pathway that leads in the direction of strategic goals articulated in advance. More detail regarding the approach can be found in two recent articles (Judge and Bauld, 2001; Judge and Mackenzie, 2002).

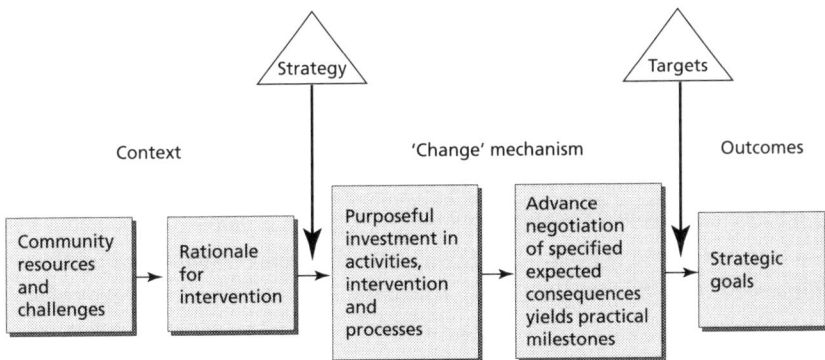

Figure 1: Realistic evaluation and theories of change: community health improvement process

Implications for local evaluation

The national evaluation has argued that the process of generating and communicating lessons about what has worked in what circumstances is a dual one. It relies not only on the evidence gathered by researchers at a national level but is dependent on the establishment of robust local processes and structures which work to embed *evaluability* in the implementation of the HAZ initiative. It is for this reason that the team has strongly recommended the use of theory-based approaches at a local level, and many of the chapters in this section discuss the usefulness of the approach in building evaluation skills and learning lessons locally.

This foreword does not attempt to capture the various components of the national evaluation beyond giving the broad theoretical background to the approach that has been adopted. At a general level, however, across the individual strands of the evaluation there is a commitment to using local learning where possible to augment our own efforts. Partly this is a pragmatic issue, since local evaluators are better placed to obtain detailed information across a range of projects within a particular locale, but partly there is a degree to which their differing role as internal evaluators will give them a different perspective on the learning which is generated. More specifically, within one set of HAZ case studies (the set of eight integrated case studies managed by the University of Glasgow) there is a particular focus on the strategic approaches that are being taken to local learning.

The coexistence of national and local evaluation partners associated with area-based initiatives does not, however, always lead to a happy marriage, and there are instances of duplication, competing agendas and antithetical approaches (Biott and Cook, 2000). It is argued that the adoption of a specified theoretical framework to evaluation at a national level that individual HAZs can *opt* to use at a local level can partially resolve some of these problems. The approach is open, after all, to building an understanding of *what works in what circumstances* at a number of levels, and legitimises the place of local learning in influencing both national and local policy development. This concurs with the view of Sanderson (2000), who argues for a greater understanding of how learning from local and national perspectives can be in competition. This process is supported by a local/national HAZ evaluation network, which has an e-mail discussion list and regular conferences. The chapters from this book have been drawn from participants at the 2001 local/national HAZ evaluation conference in Wakefield.

Learning from local evaluation of HAZs: key messages

The chapters within this section bring to light a range of issues related to generating learning from the HAZ initiative, from broad concepts about adopting theory-based approaches, to issues arising from specific evaluations of HAZ projects and programmes, and the factors impacting on the implementation of learning. By adopting a range of methods and approaches in different areas and contexts there are many unfolding stories and key messages arising. The papers highlight the potential for local and national evaluations to work together and complement each other in taking lessons forward. The evaluation of HAZs at all levels is in a strong position to contribute to the future development of policy and similar initiatives. The importance of dissemination of these lessons and examples of good practice is discussed in some of the following chapters, and is an issue that should be emphasised for any evaluation. This way, important lessons can be transferred within and between organisations for the improvement of future practice.

Theory-based evaluation

The first two chapters in this section discuss some of the broad issues in relation to adopting theory-based approaches to evaluation. Lesley Cotterill (Chapter 8) critically examines the process of developing capacity for theory-based evaluation within Plymouth HAZ, by focusing on the work of the Learning Communities Project (LCP). Although the author expresses the view that the use of a theory-based approach is helpful, for instance through sharpening project aims; strengthening links between aims, activities and outcomes; and understanding the underlying mechanisms, a number of issues about 'developing capacity' are raised. In light of the conclusion that the LCP did not 'work' as intended, and many HAZ projects and programmes have not engaged in developing evaluation capacity, this learning is presented as a set of key issues which have wider relevance to other policy initiatives.

Claire Holden and Anna Downie (Chapter 9) present some of the lessons learned from observations and experiences of the evaluation process in Sheffield and Leeds HAZs. In these two HAZs the evaluation role not only provided dedicated support to projects, but was also a mechanism of change that promoted and developed a systematic way of working. The key argument presented is that evaluation can be fully integrated into the HAZ process. However, for this to happen it requires its own theoretical basis, something which can be offered by adopting theories of change. The dual aspect of evaluation – both as a facilitator of change but also independent of it – is discussed in terms of its benefits and also its potential challenges.

Applying theory in local contexts

The chapters by Brian Jacobs et al. and Jane Springett and Angela Young offer more insight into the application of theories of change at local levels. Chapter 10 illustrates how applying a theories of change approach can enable HAZs to recognise that there are many different ideas about how communities can get 'involved' and how local people can take part in initiatives that develop community capacity. The paper argues that a key requirement is taking into account the different cultural settings that condition top-down and bottom-up approaches to community involvement. A number of local projects have been selected which show different forms or levels of activity that are considered important in building up a picture of best practice in diverse settings. The use of this approach is regarded as helpful in enabling evaluators to begin to establish what is happening in specific projects and the conditions that lead to success, without being prescriptive.

Similarly, Springett and Young (Chapter 11) illustrate the potential benefits of using a range of approaches, and show how they can be adapted locally to generate learning and build capacity within the community for evaluation. Adopting theories of change enabled links to be made at policy and programme levels, as well as encouraging rigour in planning and making the context explicit to all those involved.

Other evaluation frameworks

The third group of papers in this section explores other research frameworks that have been used to generate learning in a local setting. These chapters illustrate the application of established methods of research and evaluation in local settings and how these approaches can be adapted within the context of individual communities and working groups. Cave et al. (Chapter 12) discuss the issues around developing a meaningful approach to health impact assessment (HIA) for those individuals involved in regeneration projects who have little or no experience of public health or HIA. Having developed practical guides to assist the development of capacity for HIA in regeneration projects, the authors emphasise the importance of presenting evidence in a way that is accessible to and understood by all those involved in a project. This emphasis on an inclusive process is echoed in chapters looking at collaboration and integration in evaluation (Madeleine Murtagh) and social capital (Brigid Kane).

Murtagh (Chapter 13) reflects on the challenges and successes of this participatory approach. The programme discussed uses multiple methods of evaluation as a way of ensuring that sufficient attention is drawn to local and specific aspects of projects, and this in turn will produce more effective evaluation. The approaches used have a focus on collaboration, support and building capacity in communities and workers for this kind of work in future practice. Building capacity is also one of the lessons emerging from Brigid Kane's chapter on social capital in the South Yorkshire coalfields (Chapter 14). Local people were trained to undertake survey work and from this gained qualifications, thereby building capacity for future work in the community.

Practical lessons

The importance of taking forward the learning from evaluation cannot be overemphasised, hence the appropriateness of the title of Dara Coppel's paper, 'Learning from theory-driven evaluations across local Health Action Zone initiatives in Nottingham: using or losing?' (Chapter 15). The aim of theory-based evaluation is that of influencing policy and policy refinement; evaluation research is often used in a conceptual rather than an instrumental way, and evaluators need to increase efforts to get their message heard and to communicate the best information. Coppel explores how effective Nottingham HAZ has been in maximising the application of learning and new behaviour to core activities of organisations and policies, and assesses whether this approach in providing evidence has been useful and acceptable to local service decision-makers and policy makers. The importance of identifying what works best in specific circumstances is emphasised and illustrated by an example from Nottingham – frontline staff were given the opportunity to carry out research which increased their capacity to undertake evaluation and influence service delivery. There is an obvious role for evaluation in influencing government policy making. HAZs cannot afford to sit on the results, citing the difficulties of the initiative, inadequacy of resources and changing priorities. The learning from evaluation needs to make a contribution in raising new issues and altering the nature and climate of discussions.

Contribution of learning to the wider agenda

It is of vital importance therefore that any evaluation of Health Action Zones makes a significant contribution to the learning that HAZs have the potential to generate. Evaluation can contribute to this learning in a variety of ways, but perhaps most importantly through helping HAZs put substantial effort into developing the strongest possible rationales for the investments that they choose to make. This implies a new role for evaluators that has an important developmental element, and involves close and consistent contact with stakeholders. A theory of change approach can be blended together with realistic evaluation to provide a theoretically informed framework that will assist these stakeholders in developing rationales for action, as well as providing a framework within which evidence of change can be demonstrated.

As discussed earlier, it may be useful for a national evaluation to provide a framework that local areas can opt to use. It is clear that this approach has been useful in some instances, and the framework used by the national evaluation team (see Figure 1) has been adapted to local circumstances and developed in relation to specific projects. However, this chapter also serves to highlight the use of a wider range of evaluation activities and research frameworks, and their importance in the contribution to learning from Health Action Zones.

A number of innovative approaches to learning are demonstrated in the following chapters. Innovative approaches have been used to build capacity for more theoretical and traditional evaluation methods before a wider audience. In doing this evaluation has been made more accessible. By training local community members to become evaluators, ownership of many projects is increased and communities are empowered by the process. Another benefit is that the lessons learned from this process become part of the community resources available to refine and develop the health improvement process in the future.

The potential to generate learning from Health Action Zones has been demonstrated by projects and programmes across the different HAZs. This learning has come from a wide range of complex activities that have provided significant challenges from which individuals and organisations have drawn some important lessons. Some of these lessons are reflected in the chapters that follow.

References

Biott, C. and Cook, T. (2000) 'Local evaluation in a national early years excellence centres pilot programme: integrating performance management and participatory evaluation', *Evaluation*, 6/4, 399–413.

Connell, J. P. and Kubisch, A. C. (1998) 'Applying a theory of change approach to the evaluation of comprehensive community initiatives: progress, prospects, and problems', in Fulbright-Anderson, K., Kubisch, A. C. and Connell, J. P. (eds) *New approaches to evaluating community initiatives*, vol. 2, *Theory, measurement, and analysis*, Washington, DC: The Aspen Institute.

Judge, K. and Bauld, L. (2001) 'Strong theory, flexible methods: evaluating complex community-based initiatives', *Critical Public Health*, 11/1, 19–38.

Judge, K. and Mackenzie, M. (2002) 'Theory-based approaches to evaluating complex community-based initiatives', in Makenbach, J. and Bakker, M. (eds) *Reducing inequalities in health: a European perspective*, Routledge (in press).

Sanderson, I. (2000) 'Evaluation in complex policy systems', *Evaluation*, 6/4, 433–54.

CHAPTER 8

Developing capacity for theory-based evaluation

Lesley Cotterill

Introduction

Developing capacity for evaluation has been one of the cornerstones of evaluation within Plymouth Health Action Zone (HAZ). This chapter is based on the experiences of developing capacity for theory-based evaluation in Plymouth through the Learning Communities Project (LCP).[1] The learning from that project is used to discuss several broad themes:

- the usefulness of a theory-based approach to evaluation for learning about change and developing capacity
- the need to contextualise the process of developing capacity for evaluation in order to understand how factors in that context may facilitate or impede change
- the need to address issues of power and responsibility in the capacity-building process
- what counts as 'learning' from HAZs, and how 'learning' is linked to 'evaluation'.

The chapter begins with a brief overview of the theory-based approach to evaluation. Then, the LCP is described and discussed in the context of Plymouth HAZ. Next, the usefulness of adopting a theory-based approach to evaluation is critically examined. The chapter is concluded with key issues concerning developing capacity for evaluation based on a critical appraisal of that process in Plymouth.

---

[1] In the second phase of the LCP, the focus has shifted away from developing capacity for evaluation towards conducting theory-based evaluation.

Theory-based evaluation

Learning from HAZs is part of the rationale for their development. HAZs are supposed to be 'learning initiatives' and act as 'test-beds' for innovative approaches to tackling health inequalities, modernising services and developing partnership working (DoH, 1997a,b; Secretary of State for Social Security, 1999). However, building an evidence base on the learning from such complex community initiatives poses several challenges to the traditional approach to evaluation using the experimental model. Many of the features of HAZs mean that achieving experimental control is difficult, if not impossible. HAZs were introduced into already crowded contexts alongside initiatives with similar goals and target populations. HAZs cover large geographical areas, and their pro-grammes of work are hard to define or to hold constant. Further, the de-con-textualised evidence produced through experimentation does not contain an explanation of how and why initiatives 'work' or not, and it is this kind of under-standing that is needed to build an evidence base for health and social care (for fuller discussion, see Pawson and Tilley, 1994, 1997; Davies et al., 2000; Judge, 2000; Judge and Bauld, 2001; Cotterill, 2001).

The HAZ National Evaluation Team has identified the combined approach of theories of change and realistic evaluation for the national and local evalua-tion of HAZs (HAZ National Evaluation Team, 1999; Judge, 2000). The limi-tations of the traditional approach to evaluation were instrumental in the development of the theories of change approach in America. Theories of change have been described as 'a systematic and cumulative study of the links between activities, outcomes and contexts of the initiative' (Connell and Kubisch, 1998) and as 'a theory of how and why an initiative works' (Weiss, 1995). Realistic evaluation, also a theory-based approach, views the task for evaluation as 'to understand how programmes enter the reasoning of people who act and make choices in the world and change things... [It is about] changing hearts and minds' (Pawson and Tilley, 1997).

Combining these two approaches offers a way to 'look inside' the contexts within which social programmes and projects are located, and in which they expect to have their effects, in order to understand how change happens. Theory-based evaluation starts from the ideas that underpin projects. Although some information may be available in the form of project documentation, the reasons behind a project, and why it is expected to 'work', are usually contained in people's heads. Theory-based evaluation, therefore, requires close working with project leads and others to 'surface' their theories of change and to identify the underlying causal mechanisms that the project aims to 'trigger' in the local context. Working with people to structure their activities around a clear plan in which aims, activities and outcomes are coherently linked, and where the assumptions on which the project depends have been examined, sharpens project planning and traces a causal pathway for the project. This pathway can then be used to design an appropriate evaluation that tests the ideas and assumptions in context. The theory or theories of change are described in terms of context–mechanism–outcome configurations (see Weiss, 1995; Pawson and Tilley, 1997; Connell and Kubisch, 1998). Although this vocabulary sounds off-putting, it can be translated into everyday questions that project participants can pose themselves about their plans. For example: what is the project about, why is it needed, who is it for, what are its aims, how will it achieve its aims, and so on.

The context of the Learning Communities Project

The LCP is a three-year project that began in May 2000 with a remit to develop capacity for theory-based evaluation within Plymouth HAZ in a sustainable way. A budget of £60,000 was attached to the LCP to support evaluation. The project draws on several crosscutting themes within the national policy context, most notably the commitment to develop evidence-based health and social care policy and practice.

Other policy themes with which the LCP is consistent include:

• the need to introduce culture change into public services
• the importance of developing sustainable initiatives
• the shift towards empowering local people and communities.

The local context of Plymouth is one characterised by high levels of deprivation and disadvantage in several wards of the city. As a result, Plymouth hosts a range of area-based initiatives, and has achieved 'super zone' status (OPM, 2000).

However, other features of the local context in which the LCP was expected to make a difference were identified in its preliminary report (Cotterill, 2000). These included:

• a lack of clarity about the overall aims of the HAZ
• confusion about the difference between 'doing evaluation' and 'being evaluated'
• some hostility towards the Evaluation and Research Programme Board and its use of resources.

These issues were incorporated into a plan of action for the LCP. The assumptions underpinning the project at its outset were that:

• people wanted their capacity developed

- an accurate list of HAZ projects with basic contact details existed
- HAZ projects and programmes were required to evaluate their work
- a theory-based approach to evaluation had been agreed
- learning and evaluation were linked.

During the first 18 months of the LCP, all of these assumptions were revealed to be either incorrect or questionable. The HAZ team has since responded to some of these points as issues for development, e.g. by improving communication within the HAZ. Unfortunately, other issues have been addressed in a way that has cut across the work of the LCP, e.g. the development of the HAZ Project Guide (see below).

Developing learning communities

The LCP plan of action described a rolling programme of activities to educate, train and support HAZ partners in designing and implementing their evaluations; develop information systems for monitoring progress and quality, and sharing the learning; and devolve the LCP budget to support evaluation. Putting that plan into action involved:

- developing a monitoring and evaluation form
- providing introductory educational sessions about theories of change and realistic evaluation
- offering follow-up support sessions to programme boards to build on the introductory learning
- providing optional methods sessions
- planning to recruit and train an advisory panel
- setting up a database of HAZ project information.

Improving information

To address the lack of a paper chase and improve the HAZ information systems, a monitoring and evaluation form was designed with help from another HAZ,[2] with plans to develop a database of HAZ project information. To introduce the LCP and dispel some of the confusion about doing evaluation, an article was prepared for inclusion in the *HAZ Bulletin*. To clarify whether there was a requirement for evaluation, the HAZ Chairs Group were asked to make a decision. They decided that all HAZ projects were required to conduct evaluations and to complete a monitoring and evaluation form. However, the timescale for

---

[2] Thanks are due to Dara Coppel, Nottingham HAZ.

implementing the LCP plan was constrained by two factors: the need to allocate the LCP budget before the end of the financial year, and the deadline set by the HAZ Chairs Group for the return of LCP forms, some six weeks after the LCP introductory sessions.

Providing training

The introductory educational sessions were designed as two interlinked full-day sessions that were repeated to provide alternative dates. The first session was an introduction to theories of change, and the second, an introduction to realistic evaluation. The monitoring and evaluation form was structured in terms of the theory-based approach, and included a section asking for basic project information, and a section for requests for financial support. The format and purpose of these forms were explained at the introductory sessions, and participants were given the opportunity to draft an outline theory of change in the first session, and then use it to plan their evaluation in the second session. Participants also had time to learn about what other people were doing in the HAZ, and to discuss where their project fitted into delivering the aims of the HAZ.

Devolving the budget

To allay concerns about the use of the LCP budget, and to provide another opportunity to develop capacity for evaluation, a system was devised whereby a mixed group of people would be recruited to an advisory panel. This panel would assess project plans for evaluation, provide feedback for development and make decisions about how the budget should be allocated to support evaluation. This system was also intended to be a quality control mechanism. All participants of the LCP sessions were given the opportunity to become part of this panel, and terms of reference were developed. Originally, a succession of panels was envisaged that would enable a larger number of people to develop their skills in critically appraising evaluation designs and generating feedback for development. However, the time constraints associated with devolving the LCP budget meant that only one Panel could be trained.

Monitoring LCP outcomes

The article for the *HAZ Bulletin* was never published. People who attended the LCP training events provided very positive feedback, but the numbers were low. Replies to invitations indicated that busy diaries and annual leave accounted for some of this poor attendance, with some people commenting that allocating two full days to such training was unrealistic for them. Therefore, a series of short sessions was offered to address these issues. While this strategy attracted more people, a number of key HAZ partners were not among those accessing the training. Follow-on tailored support sessions were offered to all programme boards on two separate occasions, with no take-up. The closing date for returning the monitoring and evaluation forms passed unheeded by the majority of programme boards and projects. Only 10 out of approximately 64 project forms were received by the deadline, 6 of which were incomplete and most of the remainder requiring further work. Only one application for financial support was received. Since that time a further 16 forms have been received. The HAZ Chairs Group were appraised of this situation on several occasions, but no change has resulted. The advisory panel never met because there were no applications for them to assess.

Development of a HAZ Project Guide

The development of the HAZ Project Guide in 2001 by the HAZ team, although long overdue, was done without any prior consultation with the LCP. Further, it was done in a way that, to all intents and purposes, overturned the decision of the chairs group that projects were required to return their LCP monitoring and evaluation forms. The guide uses a form that duplicates much of the information requested in the LCP form. Although this was pointed out, along with the increase in workload for project leads, and the potential for confusion, the suggestion that both purposes would be served by focusing on helping projects to complete their LCP forms was rejected. A request from the Evaluation and Research Programme Board that projects that had not returned their LCP form with details of how they intended to evaluate their work should not be included in the guide, in order to give them an incentive to meet their requirements, was also rejected. Questions about the status and proposed use of information collected for the guide under the heading 'Results/ Evaluation' revealed that this information was not intended for inclusion on the website, but for 'internal purposes' only. These 'internal purposes' turned out to include requests for information from government agencies and ministers, policy makers and so on. Given the dearth of evaluation among HAZ projects and programme boards in Plymouth, this raises issues about:

- what counts as 'evidence'
- the relationship between evaluation and 'learning' in HAZs
- the role of evaluation in building an evidence base to inform policy and practice.

Another factor in the local context that has tended to undermine the work of the LCP is the constant stream of challenges to the adoption of a theory-based approach to evaluation. Despite attempts to introduce some clarification, there has been continuing confusion about the difference between logframes and theory-based evaluation, whether logframes were required for all HAZ projects, and whether logframes could be used instead of conducting evaluation. However, even within the Evaluation and Research Programme Board, the theory-based approach to evaluation has been severely criticised on several occasions, with suggestions that the LCP should adopt a more 'robust' approach.

Changing learning communities

Close monitoring of the LCP over the first months led to changes, with more direct support being provided to projects. Feedback from projects was very positive, although the numbers of projects helped in this way was small. This was due to the time-consuming nature of the work (see Barnes et al., 2001). The LCP monitoring and evaluation form was used as the basis for direct work with projects. As argued by Weiss (1995), the LCP found that using a theory-based approach was helpful in terms of:

- sharpening project aims
- clarifying how and why the project activities were expected to deliver those aims
- getting projects to specify their outcomes in the short, medium and long term
- strengthening the linkages between the aims, activities and outcomes
- understanding the underlying mechanisms through which the project expected to have its effects
- alerting projects to the type of monitoring data that must be collected in order to trace the pathways identified
- identifying appropriate methods to evaluate whether, how and why the project made a difference as intended
- building relationships with projects.

However, a number of issues about developing capacity for evaluation were also raised concerning:

- the self-selecting nature of this work and the implications of this for producing evaluation findings that are representative of the work of the HAZ overall
- the difficulty some projects have in making connections between what they are trying to achieve and how that fits into the 'bigger picture' in which they are located
- the variable extent to which projects are willing and able to invest the time and effort required to engage in the process of developing their capacity.

Further changes to the LCP have now been agreed with the HAZ Chairs Group, and most of the LCP budget has been used to appoint another researcher to take forward theory-based evaluation at strategic, programme board and project levels. Members of the HAZ Chairs Group were contacted by letter to ask them who should be 'around the table' for the analysis of the strategic level of the HAZ. Only four (of twelve) replied, and only one of these suggested a name – someone who had yet to take up a post in the region. Phase 2 of the LCP is now going ahead, starting with the programme board level as a 'way in' to conduct evaluation within Plymouth HAZ.

Concluding discussion

Learning from HAZs is one of the core purposes of the initiative. Developing capacity for evaluation to maximise this policy learning is consistent with the wider trends towards building evidence-based policy and practice, promoting sustainability and empowering local communities. This chapter has drawn on the experiences of the LCP project to critically examine the process of developing capacity for theory-based evaluation within Plymouth HAZ. Various factors within that local context had the effect of either blocking or undermining the process. Prior to the LCP, the Evaluation and Research Programme Board discussed at length whether a focus on developing capacity for evaluation would 'work' in Plymouth. However, insufficient attention was paid to the assumptions on which the project was based, and the mechanisms through which the LCP was supposed to have its effects in Plymouth were not articulated. A lot of thought was given to the contribution to developing capacity for evaluation among HAZ partners that other projects would make by providing resources, such as the Data Processing project. The need for a supportive infrastructure within Plymouth HAZ and the political will to make the project a success were taken for granted, rather than critically appraised. The late start of the project did not help, and it may have been, as Joan Higgins (1998) remarks, 'asking for trouble' in a context characterised by confusion and dissent.

Despite some positive learning experiences within the LCP, the conclusion has to be that the project did not 'work' as intended, and the majority of HAZ programmes and projects in Plymouth have not engaged in developing their capacity for evaluation. The learning from the LCP is presented here as a set of key issues. These key issues have relevance to other policy initiatives in which 'developing capacity' is a goal, and concern the need to recognise the following.

- 'Developing capacity' is a social process that cannot be de-contextualised. It is a process that is located in specific and dynamic social and political contexts. As such it requires critical appraisal and 'theorising' in its own right in order to make explicit the underlying assumption base, the influence of contextual factors on the success of the process, and the implications of this for achieving policy goals.

- The process of developing capacity for evaluation is flanked by a public relations agenda in which a lot depends on promoting the 'success' of the HAZs. As such, developing capacity for evaluation can be viewed as being of secondary concern to the day-to-day communications strategy for the HAZ, and may even be seen as a threat to the public face of the HAZs.

- Developing capacity for theory-based evaluation is taking place in a crowded and confusing context, in which there are increasing demands for information from the public and voluntary sectors who are required to monitor performance and adopt various accountability frameworks and mechanisms.

- Adopting a theory-based approach to developing capacity for evaluation is particularly useful in assisting projects to examine their assumptions; clarify goals; plan implementation strategies; strengthen the linkages between project aims, activities and outcomes; make explicit their ideas about how and why the project is expected to achieve its goals; and design an appropriate evaluation.

- The process of developing capacity for evaluation can, however, encounter boundary issues about who is responsible for conducting, coordinating and disseminating evaluation, as well as ensuring its quality.

- Engaging in a capacity-building process is resource-intensive for all concerned. Providing training sessions, educational materials and varying forms of 'support' may not be enough to persuade hard-pressed project leads that this is a priority. Evaluation is all too often seen as an add-on, extra work in a busy schedule, or as unnecessary in the political reality of policy making and implementation.

- The ideas of 'developing capacity for evaluation' and 'sharing the learning' from HAZs may have little in common in some HAZs. This highlights the contested status of knowledge claims in the field of social policy, and calls into question the place of evaluation in building evidence-based health and social care.

- Issues of power and responsibility tend to be unacknowledged in the process of 'developing capacity'. While such issues continue to be ignored, instead of evaluation becoming 'everybody's business' and a culture of evaluation developing, there is the danger that it becomes 'nobody's business or responsibility' if it is not seen to be in the interests of those with the power. If a de-contextualised, uncritical acceptance of 'developing capacity' goes unchallenged, it can serve the opposite agenda, with publicly funded initiatives remaining largely unaccountable, and opportunities for learning being missed.

- Developing capacity for evaluation needs to be part of the infrastructure of innovative initiatives. In the case of HAZs, developing capacity for evaluation needs to be integrated into not only its structure, but also its functioning. Developing capacity requires such an infrastructure to enable it to happen, and for its findings to be used to improve future planning and resource allocation.

- Finally, capacity building requires a realistic level of funding, and the political will locally and nationally to support such a culture change.

References

Barnes, M., Sullivan, H. and Matka, E. (2001) *Building capacity for collaboration: the national evaluation of Health Action Zones, context, strategy and capacity: initial findings from the strategic level analysis, HAZ strategic overview report*, Birmingham: University of Birmingham.

Connell, J. P. and Kubisch, A. C. (1998) 'Applying a theory of change approach to the evaluation of comprehensive community initiatives: progress, prospects, and problems', in Fulbright-Anderson, K., Kubisch, A. C. and Connell, J. P. (eds) *New approaches to evaluating community initiatives*, vol. 2, *Theory, measurement, and analysis*, Washington, DC: The Aspen Institute.

Cotterill, L. (2000) 'Preliminary report of the Learning Communities Project', submitted to Plymouth HAZ Chairs Group, Plymouth [unpublished].

Cotterill, L. (2001) 'Using theory-based evaluation to build evidence-based health and social care policy and practice', *Critical Public Health* [submitted].

Davies, H. T. O., Nutley, S. M. and Smith, P. C. (eds) (2000) *What works? Evidence-based policy and practice in public services*, London: The Policy Press.

DoH (1997a) *The new NHS: modern, dependable*, Cm 3807, London: The Stationery Office.

DoH (1997b) *Health Action Zones: invitation to bid*, EL(97)65, 30 October, Leeds: Department of Health.

HAZ National Evaluation Team (1999) *Health Action Zones: learning to make a difference. Findings from a preliminary review of Health Action Zones and proposals for a national evaluation: a report submitted to the Department of Health*, PSSRU Discussion Paper 1546, June, Canterbury: University of Kent at Canterbury [available at http://www.ukc.ac.uk/PSSRU/downloads/ddp1546.html].

Higgins, J. (1998) 'HAZs warning', *Health Service Journal*, 16 April, 24–5.

Judge, K. (2000) 'Testing evaluation to the limits: the case of English Health Action Zones', *Journal of Health Services Research*, 5/1, 3–5.

Judge, K. and Bauld, L. (2001) 'Strong theory, flexible methods: evaluating complex community-based initiatives', *Critical Public Health*, 11/1, 19–38.

OPM (2000) *The evaluation of area-based initiatives*, London: Office for Public Management.

Pawson, R. and Tilley, N. (1994) 'What works in evaluation research?', *British Journal of Criminology*, 34, 291–306.

Pawson, R. and Tilley, N. (1997) *Realistic evaluation*, London: Sage.

Secretary of State for Social Security (1999) *Opportunity for all: tackling poverty and social exclusion*, Cm 4445, London: The Stationery Office.

Weiss, C. H. (1995) 'Nothing as practical as good theory: exploring theory-based evaluation for comprehensive community initiatives for children and families', in Connell, J. P., Kubisch, A. C., Schorr, L. B. and Weiss, C. H. (eds) *New approaches to evaluating community initiatives: concepts, methods and contexts*, Washington, DC: The Aspen Institute.

CHAPTER 9

Evaluating the evaluators: the role of evaluation in Health Action Zones: some lessons learnt

Claire Holden and Anna Downie

Introduction

> Evaluation cannot afford to be too distant from the messy realism of strategy development, project design and implementation.
>
> HAZ National Evaluation Team, 1999

One of the seven underpinning principles of Health Actions Zones is that they take an evidence-based approach to their work. At a broader level, it is important to know whether HAZs are achieving their objectives and making a positive impact on reducing health inequalities (HAZnet, 2001). In this context, evaluation and Health Action Zones are inextricably linked. This is reflected in the recruitment of dedicated evaluation managers to Health Action Zones and is an innovative approach to the evaluation of area-based initiatives.

In the context of HAZs, evaluation is pragmatic in its focus, a practice-based critical review of an intervention or service that seeks to reduce the huge health divide between rich and poor. Local evaluation for HAZs was initially emphasised in order to establish how success in HAZs could be developed in non-HAZ areas (Bauld et al., 2001). As such, there is a strong emphasis in Health Action Zones on learning.

The two main strategic objectives of Health Action Zones are:

- identifying and addressing the public health needs of the local area, in particular trailblazing new ways of tackling health inequalities
- modernising services by increasing their effectiveness, efficiency and responsiveness (HAZnet, 2001).

This chapter seeks to extend these HAZ objectives into the realm of evaluation, not just evaluating how well the HAZs achieve these objectives, but how well the evaluators achieve them. The evaluation role is examined and discussed below, in the HAZ spirit of learning lessons from our work, disseminating best practice and reflecting on the progress made so far.

The HAZ approach to evaluation

The theories of change approach to evaluation (described in Connell et al., 1995) was adopted by the HAZ National Evaluation Team: this approach explores the links between the original need, the context of that need, the mechanisms of change (or intervention) to be used to tackle the problem and the final outcomes. Using theories of change as a basis this chapter looks at the context, mechanisms of change and interim outcomes for evaluation in Sheffield and Leeds Health Action Zones, as well as the lessons learnt from the management of the evaluation process.

This chapter is not based on a formal evaluation process, but on the observations and experiences of two evaluation leads and therefore the comments are not necessarily generalisable. Where relevant, the chapter will also draw on the findings reported from two universities on the basis of their independent evaluations of these two Health Action Zones.

Context

Sheffield and Leeds Health Action Zones

The 26 Health Action Zones were set up to tackle health inequalities, trailblaze new ways of working in health and social care, and modernise services. Both Sheffield and Leeds are second-wave HAZs, established in April 1999. In a city of 530,000 people, Sheffield HAZ funds approximately 40 projects, ranging from community-based 'one worker' projects to large multi-agency programmes, with particular concentrations of projects in four HAZ priority areas across the city. Leeds HAZ funded more than 80 different pieces of work in a city of 750,000 people, with a focus on improving mainstream services, alongside providing opportunities for innovative projects to tackle health inequalities (see www.haznet.org.uk for more details on the two Health Action Zones). Both Health Action Zones have dedicated evaluation posts where the performance management and monitoring role is separate from the evaluation role.

Health Action Zones: the evaluation context

Local evaluation for HAZs was initially emphasised in order to establish how success in HAZs could be developed in non-HAZ areas. In their report, *Learning to make a difference*, the Health Action Zone National Evaluation Team highlights the complexity and innovation of Health Action Zones, and the need for evaluation to take this into account: 'By and large HAZs have not chosen to implement carefully specified interventions. HAZ priorities are undergoing a continuous process of refinement that is not always clearly articulated or widely understood' (HAZ National Evaluation Team, 1999).

Reflecting this complexity, the implementation of local evaluations allowed flexibility in being able to respond to the local situation and local evaluation needs, rather than imposing a nationally defined evaluation framework. With the theories of change model as a basis, local evaluators had a relatively free hand (subject to pressures from their respective HAZ partners) to develop local solutions to the tasks of demonstrating change, and promoting and capturing learning. This reflects the ethos of HAZs in general, which allowed some freedom for local partnerships to choose the directions and priorities of the HAZ at a local level, although this emphasis on locally based solutions was diluted in the light of subsequent government requirements of HAZs to meet national priorities on cancer, heart disease and mental health, among others.

Evaluation as a mechanism of change

In both Sheffield and Leeds Health Action Zones the evaluation role was not just about providing dedicated support to disparate HAZ-funded projects. The evaluation role itself was (and is) a mechanism of change that promoted and developed a systematic way of working across the city as a whole, reflecting the HAZ way of working more widely. The evaluation support role also extended beyond HAZ into the wider health and social care community in the two cities.

In this way evaluation can contribute to the HAZ agenda, and the two HAZ strategic objectives apply as much to evaluation as to the programmes of change themselves:

- strategic objective one aims to identify and address the public health needs of the local area, and in particular pioneer new ways of tackling health inequalities (HAZnet, 2001). Addressing health needs through innovative (and therefore often untested) interventions requires thorough evaluation to assess their impact. In addition the evaluation of HAZs can provide innovative and trailblazing ways to evaluate the impact of new interventions on health inequalities.

- strategic objective two aims to modernise services by increasing their effectiveness, efficiency and responsiveness (HAZnet, 2001). Evaluation can be part of this modernisation process by providing a systematic way of assessing the effectiveness of newly modernised services.

The view of evaluation as an integral part of the innovative HAZ approach is reflected in the recent external evaluation of Sheffield HAZ, where respondents perceived evaluation and dissemination of good practice as a key theme in the innovative approach to tackling health inequalities taken by the HAZ (G. Green et al., 2001).

Just as the HAZ projects were required to provide a sound rationale for their chosen intervention, evaluation as a mechanism of change should also have a sound rationale. In order to maintain credibility, evaluation requires its own theoretical basis. In the context of the HAZ, the theories of change model provides such a basis and rationale, developing a logical pathway between context, mechanism and outcome that enables an effective and realistic evaluation to be conducted. It requires the 'theories' behind interventions to be made explicit, stating how and why activities can lead to planned outcomes. This model ties evaluation closely to project planning and project cycle management.

Therefore, evaluation as a mechanism of change is in a unique position. It has a dual role for Health Action Zones: its role as a facilitator of change makes it part of HAZ work, yet it is also independent of it. While this position has its benefits, it also has the potential for conflicts of interest. This dilemma is discussed below (see 'Organisational challenges', p. 136).

Interim outcomes: the benefits of the evaluation role

On the basis of the experience and observations of the two authors, it is expected that the evaluation process within the Health Action Zones will have achieved many benefits in the first few years of its implementation:

- A range of innovative services and interventions will have been systematically and continuously reviewed and improved, or in some cases adopted by mainstream services (using the theories of change evaluation process), contributing to the reduction of health inequalities and modernisation of services. This will build upon an underlying HAZ principle of taking an evidence-based approach to services (HAZnet, 2001).

- Workers involved in both HAZ- and non-HAZ-funded projects should have an understanding of a practical, systematic and logical approach to evaluation that is transferable to other services and settings, though this is not to say that the HAZ approach to evaluation is the only, or best, approach.

• There will be a growing body of experienced and knowledgeable evaluators who have worked in partnership with statutory and voluntary agencies and the local community to evaluate impact. In light of the changing structure of health, with power being further devolved locally to primary care trusts, these evaluators are in a unique position to build local capacity in evaluation by passing on their experiences and expertise to PCTs developing partnerships with their local communities.

• Partnerships of professionals from a variety of voluntary, statutory and community organisations should be aware of the importance of using an agreed consistent approach to the evaluation of their services.

Challenges of the evaluation role

The previous section identified several positive outcomes from the evaluation process. However, this is not to say the implementation of the HAZ evaluation process was easy and problem-free. The following section discusses some of the challenges faced during the evaluation process of the two Health Action Zones.

The challenge of project planning

The speed at which HAZ programmes were set up meant that, in some cases, the project planning cycle was truncated and project planning capacity was limited. Some project proposals were written without making a clear link between actions and outcomes.

In addition to this, an evaluation plan may not have been made explicit or costed into the main project plan, with implications for the project in terms of capacity, time and resources to undertake a comprehensive evaluation. Project planning should also have involved an assessment of the role of evaluation in the exit strategy of the project, including establishing the timescales for evaluation and to whom the outcomes of the evaluation process should be directed. In some cases, therefore, an initial revision of project plans was required before the evaluation itself could begin. Although there was often a lack of experience in project planning and evaluation, there was a desire to expand skills in these areas – the workshops run by both Health Action Zones were heavily oversubscribed.

It was argued by some that projects that are truly innovative are taking risks with a new intervention or model of service provision, and so cannot accurately define their outcomes or impact in a project plan. However, even these innovative ideas have some context and rationale, and every project needed at the very least to have a broad understanding of where it was headed. A project that is well planned and coherent is easier to evaluate effectively because it is clearer what is being done, and where the project is going. Evaluation can actually allow more innovation, as it builds in a way of assessing, reflecting and learning about new ways of working.

These initial problems in the project planning cycle were compounded by the fact that some HAZ teams were not fully in place until after the HAZ programme of projects had begun. The appointment of evaluation managers to a HAZ programme that was already established may have reinforced the misconception of the evaluation process itself as being something that comes at the end of a project and not something to be done at regular intervals throughout the life of the project.

It seemed therefore that some projects/initiatives required as much support in planning their projects as in evaluating them.

Demystifying evaluation

Evaluation of an initiative or project that is coherent and well planned may be easier, but that does not mean the evaluation inevitably yields positive outcomes for that initiative. Evaluation can be a painful process, particularly if a thorough evaluation of a new intervention or service indicates that the intervention does not have the hoped-for impact. Although painful for workers, this is as important to know as whether the intervention did have a beneficial impact and is effective, in the interests of learning lessons and improving practice. This misconception that evaluation simply grades projects as 'successes' or 'failures' underlay some of the initial anxiety and scepticism about evaluation. Evaluation can be a useful tool in promoting a culture of openness, and can contribute towards achieving the HAZ principles of equity and engaging communities and frontline staff.

In addition, evaluation was sometimes seen by projects as merely a bureaucratic exercise carried out to satisfy the funding body, and not as something of any inherent value to them. In this context, the evaluation process had to be demystified and promoted as a practical tool that could be effectively used by workers in the continuous improvement of their service. It is far more valuable for workers to view evaluation as a tool that can increase the beneficial impact of their service on the local population, and an evaluation lead can promote this view, as well as building capacity.

At the other extreme was the view that extensive evaluation was the answer, and thus there was a requirement to evaluate 'everything that moves'. However, the volume of information being collated by any one HAZ initiative can be daunting and needs to be prioritised:

> the total volume of research resource potentially available to learn about HAZs is tiny in relation to the quantity and range of activities that they represent. This implies that careful choices have to be made about how and where to focus evaluation efforts... Traditional evaluation approaches are unlikely to provide completely satisfactory ways of learning about Health Action Zones.

> HAZ National Evaluation Team, 1999

The large size of some Health Action Zones made it impractical for the evaluation lead to personally evaluate every project, so 'self evaluation' (evaluation of one's own work) was often promoted. However, there was a belief among some project workers and managers that they were not 'experts' in evaluation, and therefore not capable of evaluating the impact of their intervention. There was also concern about objectivity in relation to evaluation. Some project managers expressed anxiety that they were being required to evaluate their own service or intervention, leading to conflicts of interest.

The role of the HAZ evaluation manager therefore incorporated a 'watchdog' role, ensuring that the evaluation being conducted was as rigorous and as objective as possible. Some project managers were threatened by the implications of evaluation for the perceived value of their work. Other workers may not have previously been required to conduct such a rigorous examination of their own work. In some instances, evaluation was not taking place at all or external evaluators were being recruited at great expense to that agency. Workshops on evaluation and general project management were run for workers, enhancing their understanding and building up their capacity to evaluate.

The language and terminology associated with the theories of change approach to evaluation reinforced the perception that evaluation could only be done by experts. The theories of change framework has its own language and terminology that project managers were expected to adopt in the planning of their projects. This clashed with other agency definitions, leading to confusion about the meaning of terms such as 'outcome', 'goal' and 'targets'. Ideally, having one common framework with a common understanding of terms and definitions can reduce misunderstanding and facilitate joint project planning across agencies. While the theories of change model brought in yet another set of words, it meant that there was at least a common language that people could use across agencies.

Organisational challenges

Integrating into the health authority

There appears to have been much variation in the extent to which HAZ evaluation post-holders have been integrated into their HAZ team or health authority. As evaluation leads the two authors are located (both physically and managerially) within their health authority.

These employers (the health authorities) are one of many organisations that are subject to HAZ evaluation, which can give rise to the same conflicts of interest that some HAZ project managers reported. In other words, evaluators lose their role as a more objective observer of a system when they are located directly in it. However, being placed within the health authority also has benefits, in terms of being able to 'influence from within' and enhancing the opportunity to raise the profile of evaluation within organisations.

One way around this, as has been the case for several HAZ evaluation managers, has been to commission an external evaluation of their local HAZ, allowing the manager to provide support on an individual project basis and highlight the role of evaluation at an organisational level. This acknowledges that there are different evaluation needs for a large complex initiative such as a HAZ. Providing support and training on evaluation is as valuable a learning experience as simply evaluating the whole. This support has generally found to have been appreciated: the interim external evaluation report of Leeds HAZ found that people identified the evaluation support they had received as one of the factors that had worked well, and was felt to be successful in the Health Action Zone (J. Green et al., 2001).

In the organisational structure of the HAZ, the role of evaluation in relation to performance management was unclear. In some HAZs the roles of evaluation and performance management were separate, and in others the roles were carried out by the same individual. However, the two processes are different. Performance management attempts to answer the 'what' question: what have we done? Evaluation attempts to answer the 'so what' question: so what difference have we made? An amalgamation of the two roles may therefore send out the wrong messages about the nature of the evaluation role, and may lessen the perceived importance of the evaluation process for project managers. However, performance management is part of, and feeds directly into, evaluation, and as such the two are linked and should contribute to each other.

How much involvement?

The level of involvement of HAZ evaluation managers in individual projects also varied according to the number of projects each HAZ funds, and this has implications for the perception of evaluation. For example, in a larger HAZ an evaluation manager cannot always work closely with each project. Therefore those project managers who want to can approach the evaluation manager, while other projects choose to, or have to, work away on their own. In a smaller HAZ, projects may feel that they are being scrutinised more closely, though they may also feel they receive more support. Both approaches have their benefits and drawbacks. In both scenarios, it is important to promote evaluation as a way of working and encourage a learning culture that pervades all projects and agencies.

Good practice for the future

This chapter has used the theories of change approach to reflect on the role of evaluation. The context, mechanisms of change and outcomes have been identified for the evaluation role and the main lessons learnt thus far have been discussed, including challenges relating to project planning, demystifying evaluation and organisational challenges.

Just as we encourage HAZ-funded projects to disseminate their findings and promote good practice, so the same should be done for evaluation and the lessons we have learnt. A number of key points arise from the authors' experiences which are of relevance for future evaluation:

- Evaluation should be part of a project planning cycle of continuous reflection and action/change.
- Evaluation is difficult when a clear project plan is lacking or incomplete. Explicitly stating outcomes, activities and mechanisms is challenging but is part of good project management.
- Even when a project plan is coherent and an effective evaluation is carried out, that does not guarantee positive outcomes for an intervention.
- Evaluation is not just about being a requirement of the funding body and a bureaucratic exercise, but is of real practical benefit to professionals and service users.
- Evaluation is not the same as performance management or monitoring, although they are linked. Evaluation involves an assessment of the overall impact of a service or intervention on its target group.
- The evaluation process is a valuable resource in itself, independent of the HAZ or any funding body.

Conclusions

As we move increasingly towards multi-agency holistic strategies that tackle a host of social ills, it becomes more urgent that a consistent approach to the evaluation of those strategies and their impact on the population is used. Providing an evaluation resource to advise, coordinate, support and promote the role of evaluation is one step towards achieving this. As HAZs are becoming more integrated into local strategic partnerships they will need to consider how evaluation can be a driver for change.

The theory of change approach itself is one approach to evaluation, but not the only one. However, much can be learnt from it and its application to the work of Health Action Zones. It creates a logical pathway for planning, implementing and evaluating the impact of interventions in reducing health inequalities. More importantly, this theoretical approach does not apply just to programmes that tackle health inequalities but to a wider range of social ills, such as unemployment, crime and social isolation.

What may be of most value for organisations (whether part of a large area-based initiative or not) in which smaller projects are funded is an independent project planning support team, who could develop project planning skills with workers across different initiatives and services, incorporating evaluation into the planning process as part of the project management cycle.

However, regardless of which theoretical approach underpins evaluation, the significance of evaluation as a learning process needs to be recognised, acknowledged and built upon.

References

Bauld, L., Judge, K., Lawson, L., Mackenzie, M., Mackinnon, J. and Truman, J. (2001) *Health Action Zones in transition: progress in 2000*, Glasgow: University of Glasgow.

Connell, J. P., Kubisch, A. C., Schorr, L. B. and Weiss, C. H. (eds) (1995) *New approaches to evaluating community initiatives: concepts, methods and contexts*, Washington, DC: The Aspen Institute.

Green, G., Peters, J. and Suokas, A. (2001) 'Evaluation of the initial impact of Sheffield Health Action Zone on reducing health inequalities', Sheffield Health Action Zone [internal interim report].

Green, J., Moran, G., Percy-Smith, J. and Tilford, S. (2001) 'Thematic evaluation of Leeds Health Action Zone', Policy Research Institute, Leeds Metropolitan University [internal interim report].

HAZ National Evaluation Team (1999) *Health Action Zones: learning to make a difference. Findings from a preliminary review of Health Action Zones and proposals for a national evaluation: a report submitted to the Department of Health*, PSSRU Discussion Paper 1546, June, Canterbury: University of Kent at Canterbury [available at http://www.ukc.ac.uk/PSSRU/downloads/ddp1546.html].

HAZnet (2001) *Background: what are Health Action Zones?*, Health Development Agency [http://www.haznet.org.uk; page dated 10 October].

CHAPTER 10

Theories of change and community involvement in North Staffordshire Health Action Zone

Brian Jacobs, Susan Mulroy and Christine Sime

The aim of this chapter is to describe how we are evaluating community involvement in North Staffordshire Health Action Zone (NSHAZ) using innovative applied research to bring good practice to light. The chapter outlines our perspective and provides some examples of diverse approaches to community involvement.

We have adopted a theory of change approach recommended by the HAZ National Evaluation Team. For us, this is applied specifically to viewing community involvement. However, the community involvement aspect of our evaluation complements the larger evaluation of the NSHAZ as a whole, based on the European Foundation for Quality Management (EFQM) business excellence model.

The theory of change approach (Aspen Institute, 1997; Connell and Kubisch, 1998) enables us to research the different contexts and meanings of community involvement, and to discover innovative best practice at the local level. This is not easy as the NSHAZ is a complex partnership with 150 local level projects in urban North Staffordshire (covering Stoke-on-Trent and parts of Newcastle-under-Lyme and the Staffordshire Moorlands). The NSHAZ projects cover a wide variety of health and social issues, with community involvement being an important element in many projects. There is an Investment Group (or workstream) for Public Involvement and Community Development that aims to increase opportunities for the 'full and active participation and involvement of local people and front line staff in decisions affecting their health, quality of life and well being' (NSHAZ, 2001, 12). The group aims to stimulate innovation and learning in community involvement and in service planning and delivery.

'Community participation' and 'community involvement' imply a distinction between local people taking part in, say, consultative surveys (constituting a form of limited involvement) and people becoming actively engaged in the process of change and assuming responsibilities as part of a deeper level of participation. It is also possible to distinguish 'patient involvement' and 'community involvement', implying different stakeholder experiences. There are structured 'top-down' modes of involvement and 'bottom-up' approaches. It is therefore often difficult to define precisely what community involvement means to different stakeholders and how to evaluate local projects in terms of measurable outcomes. Community involvement means different things to different people and organisations, and as Chambers (2000, 2001) shows, the notion of 'involvement' for patients and the public is a wide one in official policy. Given the lack of clear definition of the term community involvement, and the diversity of approaches that come under the heading, it is not surprising that there is uncertainty as to how to go about assessing the outcomes of community interventions.

We have adopted a theory of change evaluation precisely because of the variety of policies and meanings surrounding 'community involvement'. We recognise that there are many theories about how change takes place by involving patients and the public to various degrees and in many ways.

The chapter shows how our approach has involved us at an early stage of:

- assessing the contexts of community involvement
- 'surfacing' theories of change for community involvement
- discovering best practice and innovation in community involvement.

Assessing the contexts of community involvement

Our version of the theory of change enables us to recognise that there are many different ideas about how communities can get 'involved'. There are many different theories about how local people can take part in initiatives that develop community capacity. By understanding the influences on community involvement, it should be possible in the future to arrive at a broader agreement about what community involvement means, using the exchange of ideas and lessons derived from different experiences.

We start by describing the cultural contexts within which local initiatives operate. A cultural perspective helps to organise our thinking about community involvement within a more coherent framework that goes some way to explain diversity and the differences of meaning ascribed to community involvement. In North Staffordshire, as elsewhere, it is inappropriate to view the working of the HAZ and local projects in terms of a single context. Different contexts reflect different assumptions and expectations about community involvement. We need to take account of the different cultural settings that condition top-down and bottom-up approaches to community involvement.

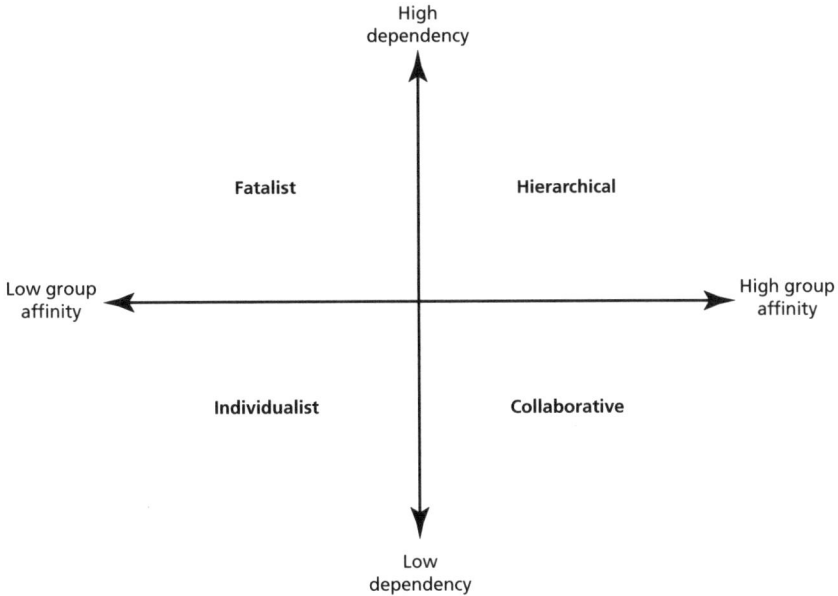

Figure 10.1: Cultural contexts

Figure 10.1 shows a grid with two dimensions that define the cultural contexts of local level projects. Thompson et al. (1990) have influenced our thinking about the grid. However, for practical exposition we have redefined the axes used in their grid. The vertical axis in our representation indicates a continuum that runs between dependency and independence. Situations in which there is high dependency are ones where local people look to others for social support – either from the state in the form of local or central government, or from the voluntary and private sectors. High dependency means that there is no confidence that people can contribute to making positive change. The further we move away from dependency, the more there is an expectation of, and culture of, 'low dependence', where people are more likely to have the opportunities to do things for themselves. This independence can translate into greater or lesser degrees of individual and/or group empowerment.

People can therefore work together to overcome dependency or they can be individually motivated. The horizontal axis in Figure 10.1 represents variations in what we term 'group affinity'. For example, on the right side of the axis, local people tend to be members of, or associated with, groups – there may be community activities organised through the churches, temples, voluntary initiatives and so on, as well as a willingness of people within the community to join various networks. The further left we move along the axis, the more 'group affinity' declines until, on the far left, there is no significant sense of group.

The grid therefore enables us to define four cultural contexts for social programmes. These are what we call the hierarchical, the fatalist, the individualist and the collaborative (see Figure 10.1). These four contexts represent combinations of the horizontal and vertical axes – of dependency–independence and high and low group affinity.

Hierarchical contexts are ones in which public and private bodies play a large part in providing and managing services in a top-down fashion within a system of supports. It is not just government that develops such supports – voluntary organisations, trade unions, the churches, schools and the wider network of private sector organisations also often provide top-down services. In this context, there is an expectation in the community that 'others will provide', or that there is a safety net provided by the state or the voluntary or private sector. Community involvement in this context is on a top-down basis of consultation and formal committee representation. In such situations, therefore, there can be relatively high organisation at the local level, especially where there is membership of local organisations such as clubs, church groups and so on, but where there is top-down provision communities as a whole are not extensively involved in decision making.

A culture of fatalism is one where there is a presumption that others will provide support services and where there is a low presumption of group affinity or community involvement. In fatalist cultures, community organisations play a small part and there are few empowering networks – there is low social capital, but still a perception that others, presumably the state or other provider, will ensure social safety nets. People have low expectations that circumstances can change for the better. They feel that there is little point in joining community associations to bring about improvements to everyday life, and they thus become increasingly disengaged and socially excluded.

The individualist context is one where people work more to their own agendas, free from the constraints of dependency on public agencies and government. This context resembles a form of individual entrepreneurialism where there is limited reference to community-based enterprise and support structures, and a greater stress on individual effort, risk taking and achievement.

By contrast, the collaborative context is strong on group affinity and fosters a dependency-reduced culture by extending collaboration and community-based enterprise. While the collaborative culture can be enterprising and even entrepreneurial, it is nevertheless one where local groups and communities work together to increase their capacities, and drive social and economic change. It is the culture most appropriate when we talk about fostering community involvement and partnership.

Surfacing theories of change for community involvement

These contexts are important because they influence the ways organisations and individuals view issues and approach community involvement. However, it is important to recognise that in practice the four cultures are not mutually exclusive. Hierarchical and fatalist attitudes often exist alongside local efforts at collaboration. The mechanisms designed to facilitate the involvement of communities combine in complex ways.

Pawson and Tilley (1997) view cultural contexts and the institutional aspects of context. For them, there is a relationship between the context, mechanism and outcomes in local projects – the 'operation of a mechanism is always contingent on context' (p. 216). This 'realistic' view of context, mechanism and outcome is, according to the HAZ National Evaluation Team, consistent with the theory of change.

For example, with hierarchical contexts there is usually an implicit expectation of dependency in a project producing a top-down delivery mechanism where local people have limited opportunities to influence priorities. One mechanism associated with hierarchy might be only the partial and formalistic involvement of the community that restricts local policy choices. The consequent outcome will likely be a neglect of community needs.

One alternative to this theory of change is where project stakeholders bring about a cultural change with local interventions based on a more collaborative approach with greater attention to local needs. We would then expect a collaborative mechanism more conducive to interventions based on partnership and extensive community engagement. A successful mechanism of this type should produce outcomes more favourable for the community even if the overall context provides barriers to success. The theory of change is then one in which local people and local organisations seek to change conditions by establishing new working relationships based on local effort and the expansion of community capacities.

Beneficial community-focused outcomes therefore are possible even when collaborative projects exist within wider hierarchical contexts. Paul Brickell (2000) highlights the problems confronted when local organisations attempt to achieve greater community involvement when central government policies contain many hierarchical assumptions. Brickell argues that all too often the result is what he calls 'communities in committee', where local groups and individuals may take part in projects, but through bureaucratic processes that limit wider involvement. Brickell argues that communities can be involved to effect change to their benefit, despite the top-down policies of government. Brickell's 'communities in business' represent an alternative to bureaucratic and over-formal structures, as they combine local social entrepreneurial initiative with collaboration. Communities in business thus represent a preferable theory of change to hierarchy and fatalism. Communities in business involve local people directly and develop innovative ways of getting things done. Local people assume practical responsibilities for improving the quality of their lives and the condition of communities.

Discovering best practice and innovation in community involvement

We have initially selected local HAZ projects where we are seeking evidence of collaboration that may advance some way towards communities in business or that develop other partnership models. The projects initially selected show different forms of involvement and levels of activity. They are projects where we suspect there may be good practice in the area of community involvement. Our view is that to display 'good practice', projects will have effective leadership, clear strategies and value-adding processes, and will be able to verify measurable beneficial results.

The following projects are of interest because they empower people by increasing their opportunities to assume responsibilities for their futures – as opposed to increasing committee work. We could have studied other projects, but these provide us with a useful early indication of the kinds of innovative activities in HAZ community-focused projects.

Advice Services in Primary Care Settings

A requirement for effective community involvement is that people should have information about their rights and opportunities for providing support for others. The Stoke-on-Trent Citizens Advice Bureau (CAB) provides advice surgeries and takes referrals from health care professionals. The advice services project provides a foundation for individuals and families in North Staffordshire to take better care of themselves and others, and to deal more effectively with the range of social and financial problems they confront. The project aims to ensure that individuals do not suffer through a lack of knowledge of their rights. It highlights the responsibilities of the services available to people, and helps overcome the inability of people to express their needs effectively.

The project employs an advice worker offering comprehensive advice on issues that may have an influence on individual health. For example, benefit advice can improve the living standard of an individual, while debt or housing advice may relieve stress.

Community involvement mechanism

The project involves stakeholders, including service users and primary care teams. Advice workers, CAB staff, primary care groups, and other health and social care professionals are included. Working with these professionals, the advice worker provides information and advice on social provisions that may not be easily accessible to local people.

There is a strong input from the CAB, which supports monitoring and reporting systems. Consultation of users in the evaluation of the project takes the form of an annual user survey. There is effective communication and support from health and social care professionals.

Outcomes

Project managers report that the project has led to the alleviation of stress-related illness, benefits for GPs, the empowerment of individual patients, increased user involvement in achieving positive health outcomes and an improved quality of life for patients. There is recognition of the importance of expanding service-user involvement, and evidence to suggest positive results along with a broadening partnership linking with mainstream organisations.

The American Clubhouse

The American Clubhouse in Stoke-on-Trent provides social, leisure, education, training and employment opportunities for people who have experienced mental illness. The project involves people who are currently receiving support because of enduring mental illness, have a diagnosed mental illness, or who suffer from persistent major distress or psychological harm resulting from their social, family or economic circumstances.

The approach is based on a successful American concept – the first clubhouse opened in 1948 in New York. The Clubhouse is a meeting place that offers services and opportunities for service users and the public, while promoting social inclusion and a positive image of mental health.

Community involvement mechanism

Although there is an identified target group, the Clubhouse has a wide range of stakeholders. It involves service users themselves, and there is involvement from health, social and educational services supporting high-quality social and therapeutic care. Leadership is flexible, linking with the established management of the Potteries Housing Association. Priority-setting involves management and users of the Clubhouse. The quality of life of the individual in the community is improved, and the project's work encompasses the local and wider community.

Outcomes

Integration into the wider community and awareness raising are outcomes of the Clubhouse. There is broadening partnership, community involvement and linking with mainstream organisations. The project also uses a 'social functioning scale' to measure the progress of individuals. This, together with practical evidence, suggests that the life of individuals has been enhanced.

The North Staffordshire Gypsy and Traveller Project Advisory Group

The project aims to improve a range of health and welfare services for Gypsy and traveller families in North Staffordshire by reducing racism experienced, tackling health inequalities, improving opportunities for children and young people, and encouraging community involvement.

An inter-agency group includes local Citizens Advice Bureaux, Stoke-on-Trent City Council, Staffordshire County Council, North Stoke Primary Care Trust, educational institutions, and the voluntary and community sectors.

Community involvement mechanism

The project provides a range of activities and facilities to the Gypsy and traveller community. Project workers interact with a wide range of social and health care professionals, and members of the Gypsy and traveller community, to identify needs and provide relevant services. The project workers have acted with sensitivity and understanding to access the target stakeholders. Learning is a two-way process, with the wider community benefiting from a greater understanding of the travelling community, and services being offered to the travelling community being made accessible and non-intimidating.

Outcomes

The project has increased family learning and educational opportunities through confidence building and racism awareness. There is a women's advisory group, increased information for the Gypsy and traveller community, and increased access to health and social care provisions. Project managers faced with the difficulties of trying to involve a disenfranchised group of people underline the importance of community involvement.

Teenwise

Teenwise contributes to the reduction of the rate of unintended teenage pregnancies among 19-year-olds and younger in North Staffordshire. The project targets all young people, including those at risk of unplanned pregnancy, with the focus on addressing the problems of lack of education, poor understanding about sexual issues and inequality of opportunity. The project provides interactive educational programmes delivered in informal settings to raise the awareness of young people. There is active participation by young people in the development of informative material and in the identification of their needs.

Community involvement mechanism

Everyone involved with the project contributes to priority setting, which proves invaluable for the young people involved. The project opens lines of communication between teenagers, parents, teachers and professionals. The strong emphasis on the direct input of young people into the project provides the basis for youngsters to gain confidence and more effectively articulate their opinions. Giving young people a voice, and enabling them to be effective as members of the community, is crucial because it gives them a sense of ownership and control. The effects of teenage pregnancy impact on the wider community, so Teenwise achieves involvement, as one project worker puts it, 'by the sharing of power with community members who have chosen to become involved'.

Outcomes

The project has provided better information to young people about sexual behaviour and ways to reduce teenage pregnancy. It has empowered young people to make their own informed decisions, and it has increased their confidence and self-esteem. Teenwise is creating an innovative and nationally acclaimed partnership between young people and service providers, which is of benefit to the whole community. It is giving young people an opportunity to develop a sense of responsibility that would otherwise be lacking.

Conclusion

These few examples demonstrate different kinds of community involvement, all of which are important in building up a picture of best practice in diverse settings (Hiebeler et al., 1999). The projects show that local people can be significantly involved in a variety of ways that add value for them and communities, and that involvement goes beyond formal committee representation. The theory of change evaluation has enabled us to make a start at finding out what is going on in projects. It does not present prescriptions about what should or should not be done, but discovers what is working and what conditions lead to success.

References

The Aspen Institute (1997) Voices from the field: learning from the early work of comprehensive community initiatives, Washington, DC: The Aspen Institute.

Brickell, P. (2000) *People before structures: engaging communities effectively in regeneration,* London: Demos with the Community Action Network.

Chambers, R. (2000) *Involving patients and the public: how to do it better,* Abingdon, Oxon.: Radcliffe Medical Press.

Chambers, R. (2001) 'Involving patients and the public: is it worth the effort?', *Journal of the Royal Society of Medicine,* 94 (August), 375–7.

Connell, J. P. and Kubisch, A. C. (1998) 'Applying a theory of change approach to the evaluation of comprehensive community initiatives: progress, prospects, and problems', in Fulbright-Anderson, K., Kubisch, A. C. and Connell, J. P. (eds) New approaches to evaluating community initiatives, *vol. 2,* Theory, measurement, and analysis, Washington, DC: The Aspen Institute.

Hiebeler, R., Kelly, T. B. and Ketteman, C. (1999) Best practices: building your business with customer-focused solutions, Arthur Andersen, London: Simon and Schuster Ltd.

NSHAZ (2001) *Investment plan, 2002–2006,* Stoke-on-Trent: North Staffordshire HAZ.

Pawson, R. and Tilley, N. (1997) Realistic evaluation, London: Sage.

Thompson, M., Ellis, R. and Wildavsky, A. (1990) *Cultural theory,* Boulder: West View Press.

CHAPTER 11

Evaluating community-level projects: comparing theories of change and participatory approaches

Jane Springett and Angela Young

Policy makers and project leads most often view evaluation as a burden. Each funding source has its own monitoring requirements, and the provision of data for performance management – 'to feed the beast' – is seen as taking energy away from what really matters, which is taking action. Where projects have a number of funding sources the burden seems even greater. Numerical targets are set which seem unrelated to the day-to-day reality of those changes in people's lives at which the programmes and policies are aimed. Such targets do little to reflect the enormity of the task and are often required within a short space of time. The pressure to demonstrate very narrowly defined 'success' saps creative energy and can undermine the original project's purpose. Moreover, projects cannot always predict their outcomes so precisely, particularly where the aim is development based on community concerns rather than prescriptive top-down concerns.

In some ways Health Action Zones (HAZs) have been no different. Performance management has been a definitive feature of the zones, imposing rigour on monitoring activities and programmes by workstream. In addition, although HAZs were originally intended to be driven by locally defined goals drawing largely on a social model of health, NHS priorities defined by central government and based on a medical model of health were subsequently imposed. What has distinguished Health Action Zones is the impetus created by the national evaluation team. Its realistic approach to the evaluation of change and its use of a co-research model has allowed local evaluation to develop within a potentially flexible framework, the theory of change model of evaluation. So, not only have Health Action Zones provided a space for innovation to flourish in terms of action, they have also allowed experimentation in evaluation for learning, i.e. evaluation to improve rather than prove.

Two examples are Merseyside Health Action Zone (MHAZ) and the Community Programme of the Manchester, Salford and Trafford Health Action Zone (MaSTHAZ). The two zones have taken slightly different approaches to encouraging projects to evaluate. They provide a useful comparative case study in engaging hard-pressed projects in evaluation. One has followed a prescribed approach using the theory of change (ToC) framework adopted by the national evaluation team, and the other has followed a bottom-up participatory evaluation model. The MaSTHAZ Community Programme adopted the former approach for their community programme/workstream and for selected funded community projects to help them develop their own evaluation frameworks. In MHAZ, a broad principles-driven zone-wide framework included a participatory action research approach to developing project-level evaluation. In both HAZs the aim was to ensure that evaluation would generate knowledge for use locally as well as at policy level, and contribute to sustainable learning systems. This paper illustrates the projects' response to these different approaches.

The approach in Merseyside Health Action Zone

Learning and evaluation were identified as key elements in the 'making it happen' stream of the MHAZ implementation plan (MHAZ, 2000). As part of the six-monthly performance-monitoring requirements, HAZ-funded projects have been asked to provide evidence of how what they are doing contributes to the seven HAZ principles ('achieving equity, engaging communities, developing a person-centred approach to service delivery, engaging frontline staff, working in partnership, taking an evidence-based approach, taking a whole systems approach'; Cropper, 2001a). To support projects an evaluation training programme has been put in place which is currently being rolled out at all levels of the HAZ, starting at strategic level right down to community level. The training programme encourages a participatory evaluation approach with the focus on learning through evaluation.

All MHAZ work is principles-driven, and evaluation is no exception. The ToC model has not been imposed as the reporting framework for monitoring and evaluation but offered as a useful tool for developing an evaluation framework, and is referred to in the MHAZ guidance on evaluation (Cropper, 2001b). Although the performance management framework laid down by the Department of Health (DoH) initially provided the framework for local monitoring reports, this was found to be inappropriate for evaluation purposes because the targets were unrelated to local aims and objectives. The local evaluation has therefore devised a framework that supports local learning. It is one that encourages participatory evaluation while promoting a consistent approach to evaluation across the HAZ.

MHAZ is a second-wave HAZ. One of the earliest projects to be funded was a participatory evaluation of a set of HAZ/Urban Projects in Netherton, an area of Sefton Borough which is a deprived outer estate on the fringes of the Merseyside conurbation. The evaluation was spearheaded by the Netherton Partnership which itself was funded by the Single Regeneration Budget (SRB). The uniqueness of the approach was that it both provided a pilot for the implementation of good practice in evaluation within the zone, and it also brought together a set of projects for the purposes of evaluation within an area (Springett and Dunkerton, 2001). Moreover, with a view to capacity building, participants would be supported through the process with training. A list of the projects is contained in Table 11.1.

An initial day workshop took place in March 2000 and this brought the projects together for the first time. The workshop introduced a process of participatory evaluation drawing on the WHO guidance on the evaluation of health promotion (Springett, 1998; Rootman et al., 2001). Following the workshop a steering group was elected and two further two-hour meetings took place. It was during this period of initial engagement with the process of evaluation that the participants were asked to clarify their theories of change, using specially created forms based on the framework developed by the national evaluation team. (At

Table 11.1 The 12 Netherton projects

Healthy lifestyles
- Local Food Links (Netherton Feelgood Factory)
- Netherton EXCEL: Stage 2 (Sefton MBC Leisure Services Department)
- Netherton Access and Information Project (Netherton Feelgood Factory)
- Health Information Project (Sefton MBC Economic Development and Tourism Division)

Childcare linked to employment
- Netherton Childcare Agency: Stage 1 Feasibility Study (Sefton Early Years Development and Childcare Partnership)
- Netherton Out-of-School Clubs: Stage 2, Infrastructure (Netherton Out-of-School Clubs/Netherton Partnership)

Community development/support/involvement
- Neighbourhood Development Project (Sefton Council for Voluntary Service)
- Netherton Volunteer Support Project: Stage 2 (Sefton Council for Voluntary Service)
- Netherton Community Transport: Stage 2, Action Research (Netherton Partnership with Merseyside Community Transport Ltd)
- Community 2000 (Community Forum Coordinator; TREND: Trust for Regeneration and Enterprise Development)

Employability of young people
- Netherton Youth Opportunities Together: Stage 2 (Netherton Partnership in partnership with Venus Working Creatively with Young Women)
- Young Persons' Resource Centre/Mobile Digital Technology Project: Stage 2 (Venus Working Creatively with Young Women)

this point there was no MHAZ handbook or framework in place.) Projects then peer-reviewed in groups each other's ToC, and these were revised.

While some projects reported that the process had been useful there was general resistance to this approach, many finding it either too linear for the types of projects they were engaging in or too long term for short two-year projects. Some of the resistance stemmed from confusing monitoring with evaluation. When discussions started on how they were going to demonstrate the achievement of their aims and objectives, the realisation dawned that the evaluation was more than number crunching, and had real potential for creative ideas and for the collection of information through a variety of other media including video, art and celebration days. These were tools that are integral to project development, particularly with marginalised and socially excluded groups who often have a low level of literacy. It was at this point the projects took ownership of the evaluation and a creative process emerged that combined learning with doing.

Ownership was a key to change in attitude and to an ongoing emergent and iterative process of evaluation development. Bringing projects together generated a broader focus and encouraged the sharing of resources and ideas. Discussion highlighted a common concern for collecting information on confidence and self-worth, income security, quality of life and community wellbeing, although these system-level indicators have not been developed systematically across the projects.

The projects took the lead in developing both the evaluation framework and training. The training focused on success, fun and celebration as a vehicle for evaluation. Participants felt that the aim of evaluation should be to capture the 'lived experience' of the projects and their impact on people's lives. Monthly two-hour meetings enabled participants, in collaboration with others, to work through in greater depth the issues raised in the initial workshop and meetings, and to support each other in evaluation. Thus the early resistance was replaced by an enthusiasm for evaluation seen as a natural activity integral to the project, rather than a burden.

In May 2001 a celebration day was held in a marquee in the main centre of Netherton. All 12 projects had a stall/display to demonstrate their achievements and outcomes, and held activities in which people could participate. There was face painting for children, and a local artist made a collage of the day. This celebratory approach to evaluation was also followed by MHAZ as a whole. In October all the projects within the HAZ were brought together in one location for a day. The aim was to provide information on what they were doing to share with others. In the morning participants were given an opportunity to evaluate each other's projects, and in the afternoon the event was open to the general public. Participants reported that this was a very effective way to encourage them to record the process and outcomes of their work as peer pressure to demonstrate progress pro-vided the motivation to succeed (Chendo Thomas, personal communication).

The Manchester, Salford and Trafford Community Programme experience

The Community Programme is a distinct stream within the MaSTHAZ imple-mentation plan (MaSTHAZ, 1999), its main aim being to build community capacity. This HAZ is one of the national evaluation case-study sites on com-munity involvement and partnership working. The Community Programme leaders decided to use the theory of change framework for local evaluation (including the development of logframes throughout the programme) to sup-port programme management and also to devolve that approach to project level. All projects had outcome-focused agreements. A number of projects were cho-sen to take forward this approach in depth. This would enable them to develop their own theory of change and use this knowledge to develop appropriate frameworks for evaluation to generate local knowledge, as well as knowledge that could feed into the national and local evaluation. Local external evaluators were commissioned to facilitate the process. These projects are shown in Table 11.2.

Each project went through the same process. In an introductory workshop, project members explored the issue of evaluation in general and the basic ques-tions that underpin the ToC. This was followed up by other work aimed at col-lecting further information, clarifying the questions and moving toward developing a dialogue with project participants. The evaluators then drafted an initial framework and fed it back to the project. It was modified as necessary and a final version agreed. This was then available for the project to use as a

Table 11.2 Manchester, Salford and Trafford Community Programme: selected projects

Project	Purpose
Four Development Sites	Geographical areas where MaSTHAZ has concentrated its partnership working to tackle inequalities
Health Action Project	Strengthen the voluntary sector
Millennium Award Scheme	Personal development (benefiting communities) for excluded individuals in the development sites
Community Action Network	Build policy recognition and support for social enterprise
Health Through Action Fund	Fund local groups in community development action
Salford School for Social Entrepreneurs	Train and support individuals to tackle the problems of their own communities
Wythenshawe Health Strategy	Partnership of regeneration, education and health with the community, to tackle health and social issues
Two Healthy Living Centre Initiatives	Submit bid to the New Opportunities Fund

framework for evaluation. The aim of the process was to 'surface' disagreement, build ownership and encourage as far as possible participatory learning.

The evaluators found a variety of challenges as they pursued these aims. The projects varied considerably. Most were funded by a range of agencies, and HAZ monies were often provided for only one year. In some cases a detailed theory of change had already been developed as part of the monitoring process but it was found not to be owned or understood widely within the project. In other cases it was difficult to engage participants in the ToC approach, and innovative tools had to be developed to encourage that engagement.

In one case, for example, project participants found that they were unable to highlight any aspects of the context in which they were working. So in the next session the evaluators enabled them to illustrate their view of the context through a metaphor (likening the project to gardening) which they had used in discussion. A range of craft materials were provided and participants were asked to create a garden which reflected what they were doing. As participants created the garden the evaluators asked them how it illustrated the factors affecting their way of working. Thus an abstract concept was given life.

Projects also found it difficult to develop a clear notion of outcomes. The evaluators tried various attempts to move towards the notion of long-term, intermediate and short-term outcomes. Project participants even found using a wall frieze (as recommended by the Aspen Institute, the originators of the ToC approach) unhelpful in grasping the approach. A technique was devised, based on long-term creative planning and neurolinguistic programming.[1] This involved getting participants to walk to a point representing the long-term future (for example seven years' time) and then gradually walk back to points in time preceding that future point (five years, two years and the present day). At each point they were asked to discuss what they saw and what needed to be in place for what they had seen at the future time point. The combination of visioning, discussion and practical reality enabled contrasting viewpoints to be articulated, and the theory of change to be developed and elaborated upon. The ability to grasp theories of change depended very much on the skill level of project management, but this simple process made an unnatural way of thinking come alive. It has repeatedly been evaluated as one of the most useful tools to help people think outside their traditional areas in terms of planning and evaluation. In MaSTHAZ it has resulted in theories of change being used by a number of projects in applications for funding.

---

[1] Jane Springett devised this tool with help from Carole Howard of Equip Training. A fuller explanation of what the tool consists of is available from the Institute for Health, Liverpool John Moores University, 79 Tithebarn St., Liverpool.

Comparing theories of change and participatory evaluation approaches

Drawing on these experiences, we now discuss the relative merits of participatory and theories of change approaches to evaluation (and those used in more conventional evaluation) in engaging communities and projects in evaluation (see Table 11.3).

Evaluation at its best is a process of reflection whereby an assessment is made as to the value of certain actions in relation to projects, programmes or policies with a view to improvement. It is in essence a process of learning from experience. Participatory approaches to evaluation are those which attempt to involve in an evaluation all who have a stake in its outcomes, with a view to taking action and effecting change (Springett, 2001). If evaluation is going to change anything it has to be useful to, and perceived as useful by, those involved in a

Table 11.3 Differences between conventional evaluation, theories of change and participatory evaluation

	Conventional evaluation	Theories of change	Participatory evaluation
Who	• External experts	• External experts in collaboration with project staff	• Community, project staff facilitator
What	• Predetermined indicators of success, principally cost and health outcomes/gains	• People identify own indicators within a prescribed framework • Prime product is a neat ToC	• People identify their own indicators of success, which may include health outcomes and gains
How	• Focus on 'scientific objectivity' distancing evaluators from other participants • Uniform, complex procedures • Delayed, limited access to results	• External evaluators through interview and discussion • Focus on fitting the information into the framework • Uniform procedures, difficult jargon • Local involvement can be minimal • Sharing of results can be delayed	• Self evaluation • Simple methods adapted to local culture • Open, immediate sharing of results through local involvement in evaluation processes
When	• Usually on completion, sometimes also mid-term	• Preferably while planning, ideally reflected on every year • Merges monitoring and evaluation but can lead to confusion with performance management	• Merging of monitoring and evaluation, hence frequent small-scale evaluations
Why	• Accountability, usually summative, to determine if funding continues	• Make assumptions and differences explicit • Give place to context • Help policy makers and encourage reflection • Satisfy the national evaluation	• Empower local people to initiate, control and take corrective action

project or programme, whether funder, participant or project worker. The aim with participatory evaluation is an approach which encourages every voice to be heard and at the very least taken into consideration when deciding on the focus and design of the evaluation (Fawcett et al., 2001).

Participatory evaluation goes beyond just being aware of stakeholder interests, however, in that there is a joint responsibility for the evaluation by the participants, who also play an active role in the nuts and bolts of evaluation (Cousins and Earl, 1995; Robson, 2000). This approach to evaluation differs significantly from much evaluation currently to be found in the research literature. Participatory evaluation is different in that the focus is on knowledge creation in the context of practice, to encourage the development of local theory, and to capacity build to encourage local learning and development (Garanta, 1993). Such a perspective is based on a completely different conception of the relationship between science, knowledge, learning, and action from that found in positivist methods in social science. It assumes that people can generate knowledge as partners in a systematic inquiry process based on their own categories and frameworks. It creates active support for the results of the process of inquiry and therefore greater commitment to change, as well as the greater likelihood that ideas will be diffused and more people will learn from them.

The aim of participatory evaluation is to make change and to teach a self-generating and self-maintaining process which continues after the evaluator/ researcher has left. The essence of this type of evaluation is that it is an emergent process controlled by local conditions (Wallerstein, 1999). Participatory evaluation is potentially empowering. It encourages innovation and change. Traditional evaluation approaches can easily undermine innovation. As people become aware of being judged they perform to satisfy the measurement chosen, instead of improving capability. The intrinsic motivation that drives learning and creates change is replaced by a desire to provide numbers for bureaucrats (Henkel, 1991; Seddon, 2000).

The strength of participatory evaluation is that it integrates evaluation into project work, allowing a more natural emerging and evolving approach to the development of aims and objectives (Springett and Leavey, 1995). It is not outcomes-driven. Rather, it plays a key role in consciousness raising. In particular it allows non-traditional approaches to data collection. But it has many weaknesses too. Participants can get so carried away with the notion of having fun that it can lack rigour and, without some structure provided by an external facilitator, direction can be lost. Too often there is a tendency to lose sight of the bigger picture. In the Netherton example, projects easily fell back into evaluating their own project rather than looking for common themes across the projects (Springett and Dunkerton, 2001). Also, unless a special effort is made, there is no feedback loop into policy structures and decision-making leading to broader changes in the policy context (Winje and Hewell, 1992).

The strength of the theories of change approach, as adopted by MaSTHAZ, is that it does provide that link with policy and programme level. It ensures the development of a framework that can be revisited by projects and programmes each year. and through which observations can be made on change. It also introduces greater rigour into project planning. Despite the struggle that both sets of projects had with the theory of change approach, individual project leads did acknowledge that it had provided them with a new way of looking at their projects. In the MaST case study the ToC approach provided future project bids with a ready-made framework for evaluation. An additional benefit was that it encouraged short-term projects to see themselves as part of a bigger picture.

There were two further great strengths of the approach. First, it encouraged the elaboration of the context in which projects were working. This enabled project participants to see what could be realistically undertaken within both resource constraints and the context in which they worked. Making explicit the context also ensured that if there were changes in the context there was an explicit framework for recording that, and ensuring that such a change was taken into account in assessing project outcomes. This encouraged recording and observation, enabling unexpected outcomes to be captured and local knowledge to be incorporated into the evaluation. The second great strength of the ToC approach was that it made the assumptions and theories of project participants explicit both to themselves and to their co-workers. In some cases this proved of great advantage in situations where there was rapid turnover of staff. More fundamentally it provided a framework for exploring and elaborating on those assumptions.

Despite these strengths, people's initial response to the whole ToC approach was that they found its language unnatural and difficult, encapsulated in jargon. They were often baffled by the rigid structure that it imposed, and much of the approach did not seem to relate to their needs. There was a sense of alienation from the evaluation as a process. In some cases it was seen as a largely academically or HAZ-driven agenda which took time and energy away from action. This lack of engagement was reflected in the difficulty in initiating meetings with the chosen projects. All in all, as the ToC originators found (Brown, 1999), using the ToC evaluation approach with community-based projects required a great deal of external facilitation.

Conclusion

To be of real use, evaluation should contribute to the development of knowledge of what works and what does not work in particular contexts and in particular conditions. It should not be undertaken in a manner that actually undermines the process and values of the projects being evaluated.

The two examples discussed here come from programmes and Health Action Zones committed to community involvement in decision making and capacity building. Building evaluation into project development in a way that encourages learning has been a key feature. Both participatory evaluation and theories of change approaches ensure evaluation is built into project planning and development in a way that conventional evaluation does not. By combining both participatory and theories of change approaches, a more people-orientated approach to targets and outcome-setting emerges, allowing those targets and outcomes to change in the light of circumstances. It has been very clear, too, that when projects determine their own theories of change, aims and objectives, the focus is not on disease and illness, which are the focus of the current national targets, but on wellbeing and quality of life, the original remit of the HAZ agenda.

It is the nature of the work of Health Action Zones that they are working with disempowered and marginalised groups. Traditional approaches to evaluation reinforce that marginalisation. Problems are often seen to be located in a particular community or group, and the evaluation often focuses exclusively on that community or group, rather than on the context in which it operates (Goodman et al., 1995). Little is done to probe the experience and assumptions of the organisations that are the source of disempowerment or to bring the two groups together in a dialogue concerning the problem, the programme, or how its success/failure will be evaluated and against whose criteria. Changing the power relations so that excluded groups can have a say and 'take control' of the factors that create health lies at the heart of many HAZ projects. The most appropriate type of evaluation, therefore, is one that involves enhancing this control (Vanderplaat, 1995). A participatory evaluation process that engages people using theories of change would have much to offer.

References

Brown, P. (1999) 'Shaping the evaluator's role in a theory of change evaluation: practitioner reflections', in Fulbright-Anderson, K., Kubisch, A. C. and Connell, J. P. (eds) *New approaches to evaluating community initiatives*, vol. 2, *Theory, measurement and analysis*, Washington, DC: The Aspen Institute [accessed at www.aspenroundtable.org/vol2/brown.htm, September 2000].

Cousins, J. B. and Earl, L. M. (eds) (1995) *Participatory evaluation in education: studies of evaluation use and organizational learning*, London: Falmer.

Cropper, A. (2001a) *Evaluation handbook for Health Action Zone funded interventions in Merseyside*, Liverpool: Merseyside Health Action Zone.

Cropper, A. (2001b) *Learning from change: an evaluation strategy for Merseyside Health Action Zone*, Liverpool: Merseyside Health Action Zone.

Fawcett, S. B., Paine-Andrews, A., Francisco, V. T., Schultz, J., Richter, K. P., Berkley Patton, J., Fisher, J. L., Lewis, R. K., Lopez, C. M., Russos, S. et al. (2001) 'Evaluating community initiatives for health and Development', in Rootman, I., Goodstadt, M., Hyndman, B., McQueen, D., Potvin, L., Springett, J. and Ziglio, E. (eds) *Evaluation in health promotion: principles and perspectives*, WHO Regional Publication, European Series, 92, Copenhagen: World Health Organization.

Garanta J. (1993) 'The powerful, the powerless and the experts: knowledge struggles in an information age', in Park, P., Brydon-Miller, M., Hall, B. and Jackson, T. (eds) *Voices of change: participatory research in the United States and Canada*, Toronto: OISE Press.

Goodman, R. M., Wheeler, F. C. and Lee, P. R. (1995) 'Evaluation of the Heart to Heart Project: lessons from a community based chronic disease prevention programme', *American Journal of Health Promotion*, 9/6, 443–55.

Henkel, M. (1991) 'The new evaluative state', *Public Administration*, 69, 121–36.

MaSTHAZ (1999) *Health through action: 1999 and beyond*, Trafford: Manchester, Salford and Trafford Health Action Zone.

MHAZ (2000) *MHAZ implementation plan*, Liverpool: Merseyside Health Action Zone.

Robson, C. (2000) *Small scale evaluation, principles and practice*, London: Sage.

Rootman, I., Goodstadt, M., Hyndman, B., McQueen, D., Potvin, L., Springett, J. and Ziglio, E. (eds) *Evaluation in health promotion: principles and perspectives*, WHO Regional Publication, European Series 92, Copenhagen: World Health Organization.

Seddon, J. (2000) 'On target to nothing', *The Observer*, 27 August, 36.

Springett, J. (1998) *Practical guidance on evaluating health promotion*, Copenhagen: World Health Organization (Europe).

Springett, J. (2001) 'Appropriate approaches for the evaluation of health promotion', *Critical Public Health*, 11/2, 139–51.

Springett, J. and Dunkerton, L. (2001) *HAZ/Netherton interim evaluation report*, Liverpool: Institute for Health, Liverpool John Moores University.

Springett, J. and Leavey, C. (1995) 'Participatory action research: the development of a paradigm: dilemmas and prospects' in Bruce, N., Springett, J., Hodgkiss, J. and Scott-Samuel, A. (eds) *Research and change in urban community health*, Aldershot: Avebury.

Vanderplaat, M. (1995) 'Beyond technique: issues in evaluating for empowerment', *Evaluation*, 1/1, 81–96.

Wallerstein, N. (1999) 'Power between evaluator and the community: research relationships with New Mexico's healthier communities', *Social Science and Medicine*, 49/1, 39–53.

Winje, G. and Hewell, H. (1992) 'Influencing public health policy through action research', *Journal of Drug Issues*, 22, 169–78.

CHAPTER 12

Predicting health change associated with urban regeneration: building capacity for health impact assessment

Ben Cave, Sarah Curtis and Sian Penner

Introduction

The East London and the City Health Action Zone (HAZ) commissioned Queen Mary, University of London (QMUL), to develop a toolkit for health impact assessment (HIA). The target audience was people working in, or affected by, regeneration programmes. QMUL aimed to develop an approach which was meaningful to people involved in urban regeneration projects and who had little experience of public health or HIA. This article describes the approach and the materials we developed (Cave and Curtis, 2001b,c; Cave et al., 2001). We explain how our approach to HIA was supported by the national HAZ programme and informed by the national evaluation of HAZ. We discuss how we introduced HIA into the context of urban regeneration schemes, and we conclude by reporting on an ongoing programme of work to disseminate these HIA materials, to integrate HIA into mainstream procedures and to develop wider capacity for, and interest in, HIA in East London.

The setting

East London and the City HAZ covers the boroughs of Tower Hamlets, Hackney, Newham and the City of London. There are great extremes of wealth and poverty within these geographical boundaries. Living and working conditions are also very variable, but on average are poor. Tower Hamlets, Hackney and Newham are among the most deprived boroughs in England; the population are young, highly mobile and contain a high proportion of people from black and ethnic minority communities. These boroughs are all within a 30 minute journey from two major global employment sites: the City of London and Docklands. East London historically plays an escalator role (Massey, 1979) within the economy of the rest of London and the South-East. It accommodates significant numbers of relatively poor people, many of them recent migrants to London, who initially find it necessary to seek work in the low-skilled sectors of the economy offering relatively poor pay and conditions. Those who manage to improve their economic position tend to move on to more affluent areas as soon as they are able. This has important implications for the planning and delivery of services, and for the quality of life of the population who remain. The mobility of the population also means it can be difficult to assess the longer-term health impact of regeneration programmes.

Background: urban regeneration and developments in HIA

Roberts (2000) defines urban regeneration as 'comprehensive and integrated vision and action which leads to the resolution of urban problems and which seeks to bring about a lasting improvement in the economic, physical and social environment of an area that has been subject to change'.

Regeneration programmes typically comprise a number of schemes which target specific geographical areas. They cater to specific local needs and they use a wide variety of measures to achieve their aims. Regeneration programmes are often made up of a number of projects which may be linked with, or going on in the same area as, other interventions. Regeneration and renewal programmes are increasingly expected to consider more than the immediate process outputs of their activities. The emphasis is now upon broader outcome measures to examine the wider effects, or impact, the programmes have on the areas and populations on which they are targeted (LGA, 1998; Government Office for London and London Development Partnership, 1999).

The health impacts of regeneration have received relatively scant attention in the past: this is partly because of a lack of accessible and sensitive indicators of population health which are relevant to regeneration (Bardsley et al., 2001). Regeneration projects have potential to affect inequalities as they are often focused on problems of social exclusion and deprivation. They act upon factors which are considered to be among the socioeconomic determinants of health, such as employment, housing and the social and physical environment of a community (Marmot and Wilkinson, 1999). Recent government guidance states that developing partnerships with sectors outside the NHS in order to tackle inequality is a key strategic role for health authorities while, across government, a high priority will be given to measures which address determinants of health (Statistics Division and Central Health Monitoring Unit, 2001; see also DoH, 2000, 2001a,b). It has also been noted that the NHS has a role to play in regeneration, as it is a major employer and consumer of goods and services (Travers et al., 2000; London Development Agency, 2001).

HIA can contribute to understanding of the links between health, health services and regeneration projects. The World Health Organization (WHO European Centre for Health Policy, 1999) define HIA as 'a combination of procedures, methods and tools by which a policy, programme or project may be judged as to its potential effects on the health of a population, and the distribution of those effects within the population'.

Key points to note from this definition are that there is no single methodology for HIA: it uses different approaches to look at a range of initiatives from policy to project level. This definition refers to *prospective* HIA which involves anticipating the likely effects of an intervention. Prospective HIA is best seen as part of planning and design of an intervention (see Figure 12.1). It is distinct from monitoring and evaluation as it comes earlier in the project cycle. Because HIA helps to identify areas where change might be expected it can feed into later monitoring and evaluation. HIA also provides a way to consider how health impacts of an intervention are distributed throughout the populations affected, and what the implications are likely to be for health inequality – HIA judges the potential for both positive and negative effects on health. On the basis of this judgement, participants in the HIA can develop recommendations as to how positive health effects can be enhanced and negative health effects reduced. Cragg (2001) discusses HIA in the context of regional strategies and states that the HIA process is an aid to, and not a substitute for, decision making. HIA provides further evidence to inform public policy: it does not dictate a solution.

There is currently a great deal of demand for HIA, and little capacity or confidence among those working in the regeneration field to carry it out. At a recent conference the WHO called for skills, tools and evidence bases to be developed in order that capacity to carry out HIA is increased (Dora, 2001). The work reported here was intended to help to build this capacity.

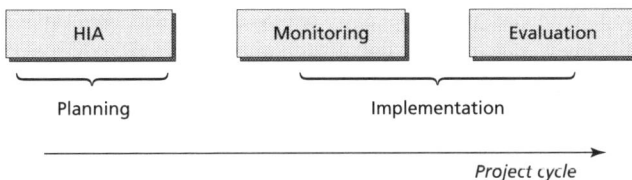

Source: Cave and Curtis, 2001b

Figure 12.1: HIA, monitoring and evaluation

The approach to HIA

The work reported here was partly funded by the Health Action Zone programme, and some of the key principles of Health Action Zones were important for developing the HIA strategies: these include cooperative work across the NHS/non-NHS interface and the emphasis on involving a wide range of partners to improve health. This initiative used the HAZ structure and funding to introduce an innovative method to organisations outside the NHS. The project reported here has produced documentation in the form of practical guides designed to assist the development of capacity for HIA in regeneration projects. Cave and Curtis (2001b) describe this approach to HIA, and show how it relates to other HIA strategies and to existing practices in regeneration. It is flexible so that the methods and approaches can be adapted to the particular project which is being assessed. We describe below how this programme of work is now looking to integrate the outcomes and lessons of this HAZ initiative into mainstream regeneration activity in the local area.

We also drew on the lessons and methods developed through the national evaluation of Health Action Zones. Box 12.1 cites the HAZ National Evaluation Team (1999), which traces similarities between complex community initiatives (CCIs) and Health Action Zones. It goes on to describe ways to evaluate the effects of CCIs by identifying the theories of change on which interventions are based. As regeneration programmes are CCIs we adapted this approach for HIA, as described below.

Figure 12.2 overleaf shows that early stages in this model of HIA involve clarifying the ways in which the context and the mechanisms of the project contribute to its expected outcomes (Pawson and Tilley, 1997). The expertise of those directly involved in the intervention is critical to identifying this CMO (context–mechanism–outcome) pattern, and we explored different ways to elicit their views, including interviews and group discussions. At this stage outcomes are not necessarily expressed in terms of health, but more usually in terms of changes to conditions in the social or physical environment, such as housing, employment or community relationships. This process of identifying the CMO pattern was familiar to staff managing the project and to stakeholders from community groups who had participated in previous consultation exercises. It was useful to take people through the process in more detail so that they could restate their aims. It was also very important that HIA could thus been seen as an extension of normal practice in the management of regeneration projects.

The next phase of the HIA process involved considering the expected regeneration outcomes in terms of their possible impacts on health. An evidence base was produced to assist this stage (Cave et al., 2001). We conducted a semi-structured review of published research evidence on the links between determinants of health and health outcomes. The review focused on evidence relating to

Box 12.1 Complex community initiatives

[The following] characteristics pose a number of important challenges for evaluators, and for the use of traditional evaluation methodologies. Both CCIs and HAZs aim to:

- promote positive changes in individual, family and community institutions
- develop a variety of mechanisms to improve social, economic and physical circumstances, services and conditions in disadvantaged communities, and
- place a strong emphasis on community building and neighbourhood empowerment.

These characteristics pose a number of challenges for evaluation, including that:

- initiatives have multiple, broad goals
- they are highly complex learning enterprises with multiple strands of activity operating at many different levels
- objectives are defined and strategies chosen to achieve goals that often change over time
- many activities and intended outcomes are difficult to measure
- units of action are complex, open systems in which it is virtually impossible to control all the variables that may influence the conduct and outcome of evaluation.

Source: HAZ National Evaluation Team, 1999, 17

selected health determinants most relevant to our regeneration case studies: housing, employment, transportation and social capital. We concentrated especially on evidence which showed how *change* in a determinant of health might affect health. In presenting the review we aimed to clarify how changes in particular aspects of health determinants were associated with change in health, and what mechanisms (or causal pathways) might explain the association. We considered how to assess different types of evidence from research. The most useful evidence came from longitudinal studies of samples of individuals, which could demonstrate these relationships most clearly. However, much of the evidence from longitudinal studies relates to the health impact of negative change in health determinants, such as experience of poor housing or redundancy and unemployment. There is a relative lack of research on what happens to people's health when the determinants of health improve. This is important for HIA of regeneration, since the expected changes to determinants of health will in many cases be positive.

Screening and scoping the project

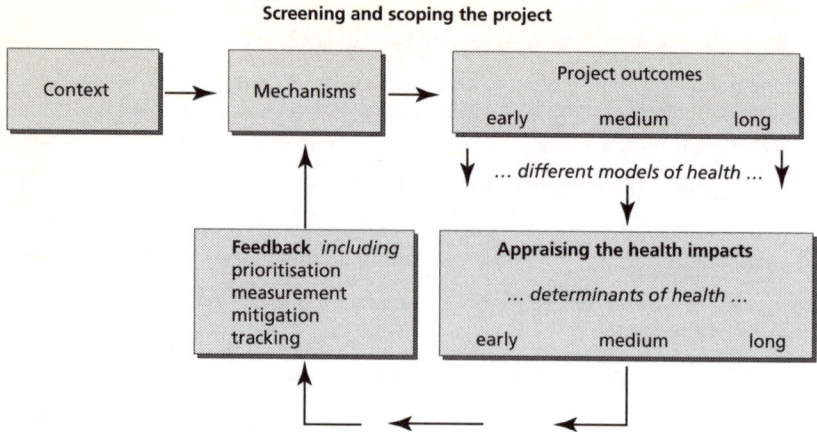

Source: Cave and Curtis, 2001b

Figure 12.2: Health impact assessment and the project cycle

Figure 12.2 also shows the last stage of HIA, which involves feeding back what has been learnt into the project decision-making process.

The general approach illustrated in Figure 12.2 was demonstrated in some case studies which are described in greater detail in Cave and Curtis (2001a,b,c) and Curtis et al. (2002, in press). Our guide to HIA outlines some key questions to consider when working through an HIA (see Box 12.2), and we illustrate here how these questions were addressed in one of the case studies.

Demonstrating HIA: learning from a case study

Building Sustainable Communities is a regeneration programme comprising several different projects. It was agreed with the programme manager and the local authority that the case study for the HIA demonstration would focus on a housing project which was a main component of the Building Sustainable Communities programme.

The first set of questions in Box 12.2 concern terms of reference and responsibilities. In order to address these, a steering or advisory group needs to be set up to agree on the strategy for HIA, provide contacts within the project, ensure continuity from the beginning to the end and ensure that the recommendations will fed into the delivery of the project. In this case study the HIA facilitator coordinated the establishment of this group. In a different situation, if project managers take the initiative to consider HIA, a facilitator might need to be appointed by the steering group.

Box 12.2 Questions to consider in HIA

Getting started

Agree terms of reference and responsibilities:
- Who is the intended audience for the recommendations from HIA?
- Who will facilitate and steer the HIA?
- How will HIA fit into the activity of the organisation planning the project?
- Who will participate in HIA?

Screening and scoping

Context:
- What are the circumstances in which the project will work?
- Where is the project operating?
- Who are the people who are likely to be involved in, or affected by, the project?
- What are the health characteristics of the local population in the project area?

Mechanism:
- How will the project work?
- Will something be done differently? If so, why?
- Will new staff come into post? If so, what will they do?
- Will new facilities be created? If so, what is their purpose?

Planned project outcomes: what will the effects of the project be in the:
- short term?
- medium term?
- long term?

Rapid appraisal of health outcomes

- Which determinants of health are likely to be affected by the project?
- How may health determinants change as a result of a project?
- How might expected changes in these determinants of health affect the health of people in the project?
- What might be the outcomes for health?

Feedback to project design

- What changes, if any, should be recommended to the project plans in the light of the rapid HIA?
- How might these changes be measured or assessed?
- How might these changes be monitored and evaluated?
- Will the stakeholders commission a more detailed HIA or an evaluation which focuses on the most important health outcomes to which they have given the highest priority?

Source: Cave and Curtis, 2001b

An early meeting between the HIA facilitator and the project manager provided a list of contacts who would be key informants. The facilitator conducted a series of interviews with the key informants and then convened a HIA workshop with a wider group, recruited from the consultation group set up for the project. In these interviews and the workshop we worked through the framework in Figure 12.2 to find answers to the questions in Box 12.2.

The interviews and the workshop established the CMO pattern for this initiative. The context is an area with significant numbers of low-quality, privately rented houses which offer poor living conditions and have high levels of multiple occupation and crowding. Most of the rent paid to the private landlords comes from housing benefit, so this has been identified as state-subsidised poor housing in need of improvement. The mechanisms for improvement set up through Building Sustainable Communities include a housing company established to oversee a programme of housing improvements and to continue after seven years of regeneration funding is finished. The housing company seeks to improve private-sector housing through a programme of refurbishment and enveloping repairs. An important part of the strategy is to encourage private landlords to register their properties with the housing company. Landlords who are on the register must maintain their properties to acceptable standards and will receive assistance in return. Compulsory purchase of properties by the housing company is a possible sanction if landlords are unwilling to join the register or to improve their properties.

The project is associated with other initiatives to improve the infrastructure in the area and promote more local employment opportunities. In terms of outcomes, key informants and workshop participants expected that the wider programme and the housing refurbishment would have long-term positive effects on the local environment and would encourage people to stay permanently in the area, creating a more stable population. It was also acknowledged that there would be variable effects for different groups of local residents. Some people who were currently living in temporary accommodation would have to move out of the area: some workshop participants were concerned that this might lead to continuing problems with homelessness.

Having established the CMO pattern, the HIA participants were encouraged to consider a rapid appraisal of potential health outcomes. This part of the HIA was informed by the review of the public health evidence base concerning links between housing and health (Cave et al., 2001). This helps participants to see expected regeneration outcomes as potential changes in health determinants: this in turn leads to an assessment of the likely health impacts of these changes. Research literature suggests that improving housing may bring long-term health benefits for those people whose living conditions are improved. The short-term health effects are less certain (see Ambrose, 1996, 2000; Ambrose et al., 1996;

Collard, 1997, 2000; Allen, 2000; Thomson et al., 2001). The evidence suggests that it is important to manage the transition phase as the building works are carried out, both for the people who remain and for those who will be rehoused elsewhere. The transition can involve physical hazards due to building activities, and psychosocial impacts of disruption and change. The refurbishment of housing will reduce the number of houses in multiple occupation (HMOs) and some residents will be displaced, especially if they cannot afford the higher rents. Therefore the scheme may not reduce health inequalities.

The feedback stage involved a presentation by the facilitator to the planning board for the Building Sustainable Communities programme. In the ensuing discussion it was recommended that the short-term risks posed by the building works could be countered with health and safety training for the contractors, and road safety training for children in the local schools. Medium-term recommendations were to prioritise the allocation of vacancies to families who are moved out of HMOs, and develop a programme of brokerage to ensure that people get the most from interactions with statutory agencies. Longer-term recommendations included action to address community development needs, so that the improvements to the physical environment are matched with improvements in the social environment. There was also a recommendation to formally involve the health sector in the delivery of the programme.

The process of HIA enabled programme managers to identify the wider effects of their work and to take a new perspective on the project. The process of constructively identifying the potential for negative effects, as well as positive effects, of housing improvement initiatives was useful, since the normal process of managing regeneration projects does not always encourage this. The programme management responded to the recommendations, and initiated a family welfare project and a drugs and alcohol project to address some of the issues raised.

Conclusions from the demonstrations and lessons for mainstream practice

Regeneration and renewal operate on determinants of health and therefore have a significant potential for changing public health. The housing example described above illustrates how evidence about the likely health effects of regeneration suggests that the changes may be beneficial to health in some ways, but that there is also potential to damage health and exacerbate existing inequalities. Prospective HIA seems necessary as a way to make the planning of regeneration schemes sensitive and responsive to these possible health impacts. This could enhance the potential of regeneration programmes to improve public health and reduce health inequalities.

Some models of HIA, such as the one adopted here, are consistent with the aims of the HAZ programme for wider involvement, as they emphasise participation of a wide range of stakeholders and community groups. HIA for regeneration requires improved coordination between the different agencies responsible for health and for regeneration. Therefore, in this example, HIA was usefully addressed through the HAZ programme, because of the emphasis in HAZ on cross-sectoral working.

HIA should be based on an ethical use of the available public health evidence. The evidence needs to be made available in a way that is relevant for regeneration schemes. It needs to be presented in forms that can be understood and interpreted by a range of stakeholders involved in regeneration, who are not likely to be specialists in public health. Both qualitative and quantitative information is relevant for HIA, and quantitative data should not necessarily be given more weight than sound qualitative evidence. The existing evidence base for HIA is not likely to provide precisely quantifiable predictions of future health impact. It is more likely to show the kinds of health impacts which might be expected from a project. Anticipating these allows them to be considered at the planning stage of a project and assessed as part of any evaluation of the project outcomes. We saw above how HIA provides information to aid decision making.

If it is to be applied effectively in the regeneration field, HIA should be integral to existing regeneration planning procedures and not a 'parallel' or 'additional' activity. The work we have described forms the basis of a continuing programme to develop wider capacity for and interest in HIA in East London. One part of the strategy has been to demonstrate through case studies that HIA is a useful planning tool, which can help with achieving wider regeneration objectives. We are also working at a strategic level with local authorities and local strategic partnerships to integrate questions about health and wellbeing into standard regeneration procedures, so that programmes which are bidding for monies will consider their potential impact on health. We are disseminating the materials produced from this HAZ initiative as widely as possible by various media, including the internet (see http://www.geog.qmul.ac.uk/health/guide.html for Cave and Curtis, 2001b,c, and Cave et al., 2001). Using the learning from the case studies, we are developing training programmes to improve the capacity for HIA in regeneration programmes in East London more generally. We acknowledge that this could be contentious. In debate at a recent HIA conference (Richards and Abrahams, 2001) many people felt that the provision of formal training programmes contradicted the democratic values of HIA as it risked professionalising the approach and so excluding those people without the necessary qualifications.

However, we believe that there is currently a great demand for HIAs and that in practice a relatively small number of expert consultants are carrying them out, which is not necessarily beneficial for democratic involvement either. Concerns about professionalisation are valid, but expanding the range of HIAs will mean that quality controls become important: organisations will not commission HIAs if they are not confident that they will be able to recognise the value of the completed work. Wider availability of training will demystify the process, show that HIA shares skills with other regeneration management techniques and empower more people to use HIA effectively. It may be important to aim to recruit trainees in HIA from the local communities where regeneration is taking place in order to enhance local capacity.

Acknowledgement

This work and its dissemination were supported by the East London and the City Health Action Zone, the Department of Health, the Drapers Fund and by Queen Mary, University of London. We thank the people in the regeneration projects who worked with us and contributed time and energy. The authors, not the supporting organisations, are responsible for the views expressed here.

References

Allen, T. (2000) 'Housing renewal: doesn't it make you sick?' *Housing Studies*, 15/3, 443–61.

Ambrose, P. (1996) *'I mustn't laugh too much': housing and health on the Limehouse Fields and Ocean Estates in Stepney. First report of Project HC4 – The 'health gain' survey*, London Borough of Tower Hamlets SRB Programme, Centre for Urban and Regional Research, University of Sussex.

Ambrose, P. (2000) *A drop in the Ocean: the health gain from the Central Stepney SRB in the context of national health inequalities*, Brighton: Health and Social Policy Research Centre, University of Brighton.

Ambrose, P., Barlow, J., Bonsey, A., Pullin, M., Donkin, V. and Randles, J. (1996) *The real cost of poor homes*, London: The Royal Institution of Chartered Surveyors, 1–62.

Bardsley, M., Cave, B., Jacobson, B. and Garvican, L. (2001) *Monitoring regeneration and health: a health indicators toolbox*, London: Health of Londoners Programme [available at http://www.holp.org].

Cave, B. and Curtis, S. (2001a) 'Developing a practical guide to assess the potential health impact of urban regeneration schemes', *Promotion and Education*, 8/1, 12–16.

Cave, B. and Curtis, S. (2001b) *Health impact assessment for regeneration* projects, vol. 1, *A practical guide*, London: East London and the City Health Action Zone and Queen Mary, University of London [available at http://www.geog.qmul.ac.uk/health/guide.html].

Cave, B. and Curtis, S. (2001c) *Health impact assessment for regeneration* projects, vol. 3, *Principles*, London: East London and the City Health Action Zone and Queen

Mary, University of London [available at
http://www.geog.qmul.ac.uk/health/guide.html].

Cave, B., Curtis, S., Coutts, A., and Aviles, M. (2001) *Health impact assessment for regeneration projects*, vol. 2, *Selected evidence base*, London: East London and the City Health Action Zone and Queen Mary, University of London [available at http://www.geog.qmul.ac.uk/health/guide.html].

Collard, A. (1997) *Settling up: towards a strategy for resettling homeless families*, London: London Homelessness Forum.

Collard, A. (2000) *Rehousing for health: making or breaking the link between housing deprivation and health inequalities? A report on the findings of the Health Gain and Medical Housing Transfer Project*, London: Tower Hamlets Health Strategy Group.

Cragg, L. (2001) *Policy-making and health impact assessment*, London Health Commission [personal communication].

Curtis, S., Cave, B. and Coutts, A. (2002) 'Is urban regeneration good for health? Perceptions and theories of the health impacts of urban change', *Environment and Planning C* [in press].

DoH (2000) *The NHS Plan: a plan for investment – a plan for reform*, Cm 4818-1, The Stationery Office [available at http://www.doh.gov.uk/nhsplan/nhsplan.htm].

DoH (2001a) *From vision to reality*, London: Department of Health [available at http://www.ohn.gov.uk/glossary/vision.pdf].

DoH (2001b) *Tackling health inequalities: consultation on a plan for delivery*, London: Department of Health [available at http://www.doh.gov.uk/healthinequalities].

Dora, C. (2001) Keynote speech, Fourth UK HIA Conference, Liverpool.

Government Office for London and London Development Partnership (1999) *Single Regeneration Budget round 6 bidding guidance: a guide for partnerships in London*, London.

LGA (1998) *New commitment to regeneration: a guidance note to pathfinders for preparing a comprehensive regeneration strategy and action plan*, London: LGA Publications [available at http://www.lga.gov.uk/lga/newcommitment/backgroundnote.pdf].

London Development Agency (2001) *Success through diversity: London's economic development strategy*, London [available at http://www.lda.gov.uk].

Marmot, M. and Wilkinson, R. G. (1999) *Social determinants of health*, Oxford: Oxford University Press.

Massey, D. (1979) 'In what sense a regional problem?', *Regional Studies*, 13, 233–43.

HAZ National Evaluation Team (1999) *Health Action Zones: learning to make a difference. Findings from a preliminary review of Health Action Zones and proposals for a national evaluation: a report submitted to the Department of Health*, PSSRU Discussion Paper 1546, June, Canterbury: University of Kent at Canterbury [available at http://www.ukc.ac.uk/PSSRU/downloads/ddp1546.html].

Pawson, R. and Tilley, N. (1997) *Realistic evaluation*, London; Thousand Oaks, California: Sage.

Richards, Z. and Abrahams, D. (2001) 'Developing a competency framework for HIA practitioners', Fourth UK HIA Conference, Liverpool.

Roberts, P. (2000) 'The evolution, definition and purpose of urban regeneration', in Roberts, P. and Sykes, H., *Urban regeneration: a handbook*, London: Sage Publications, 9–36.

Statistics Division and Central Health Monitoring Unit (2001) *Technical supplement on target setting for health improvement*, Department of Health [available at http://www.ohn.gov.uk/ohn/technical/technical].

Thomson, H., Petticrew, M. and Morrison, D. (2001) 'Health effects of housing improvement: systematic review of intervention studies', *British Medical Journal*, 323, 187–190.

Travers, T., Glaister, S. and Graham, D. (2000) *Capital asset: London's healthy contribution to jobs and services*, London: NHSE.

WHO European Centre for Health Policy (1999) *Health impact assessment: main concepts and suggested approach*, Gothenburg Consensus Paper, Brussels: WHO Regional Office for Europe, ECHP [available at http://www.who.dk/hs/ECHP/index.htm].

CHAPTER 13

Collaboration and integration in evaluation: evaluating the HAZ in Newcastle

Madeleine J. Murtagh

Introduction

Meanings and understandings of health are complex, multiple and diverse. Over the past two decades health promotion initiatives that recognise this complexity have employed a wide range of approaches, not least in strategies for tackling health inequalities. Evaluation of diverse and complex strategies for tackling health inequalities requires multiple methods, often across more than one research tradition. Appropriate evaluation also requires attention to the particular intervention and setting: to the people, project and outcomes of the project.

This chapter outlines the development and implementation of a tailored evaluation strategy, implemented in the Newcastle Division of the Tyne and Wear Health Action Zone, which aimed to be methodologically appropriate, collaborative and integrated in such a way as to contribute to the process of change embarked upon by projects addressing health inequalities. Arguably the most important learning to evolve in such circumstances arises from the challenges posed in attempts at innovation, more so than from the evident successes of the process. This chapter examines and reflects on those challenges and successes in the evaluation of the Newcastle division of the Tyne and Wear Health Action Zone (hereafter the HAZ in Newcastle).

Context

Health inequalities are now on the health policy agenda in a way that didn't seem possible just five years ago. Since the publication in the early 1980s of the Black report (Black et al., 1992) much has been written in the professional and academic literature about the causes and extent of health inequalities, but in the mid-1990s there emerged an emphasis on the need to 'do something' rather than study further the nature of the subject (Bunton and Burrows, 1994; Benzeval et al., 1995). Labour government health policies and initiatives increasingly appear to address long-standing calls to tackle health inequalities (the Acheson report, *Independent inquiry into inequalities in health*, 1998; establishment of Health Action Zones, 1998; the white paper *Saving lives: our healthier nation*, 1999; the establishment of the Health Development Agency, 2000; and publication of the *NHS Plan*, 2000, and *Tackling health inequalities: consultation on a plan for delivery*, 2001).

Emerging with an attention to health inequalities has been an increasing recognition of the capacity of individuals and communities to influence their health and health care. Current health policy, for example, stresses the importance of public and patient involvement in decision making (see, for example, the Department of Health publications *Patient and public involvement in the new NHS*, 1999; *NHS Plan*, 2000; *Shifting the balance of power within the NHS*, 2001; *Involving patients and the public in healthcare: a discussion document*, 2001; *The expert patient*, 2001).

In this context 26 Health Action Zones were established in areas of deprivation and poor health, with the express purpose of tackling health inequalities. Although the emphasis changed to accommodate NHS priorities from 2000, the stated aim of HAZs, in the invitation to bid for HAZ status, was 'to develop and implement a health strategy that cuts inequalities, and delivers within their areas measurable improvements in public health and health outcomes, and quality of treatment and care'. Health Action Zones across England developed multiple strategies to achieve this. The Tyne and Wear Health Action Zone was established as a first-wave HAZ in 1998. It covers five local authority districts with a total population of 1.1 million: Newcastle upon Tyne, North Tyneside, South Tyneside, Gateshead and Sunderland. In the HAZ in Newcastle) the Newcastle Health Partnership forms the main focal point for coordinating and steering local HAZ action. The partnership comprises a wide range of organisations within the city, including the council, health authority, hospital and primary care trusts, the Healthy City Project, local universities, the voluntary sector, the police and community members.

The work of the HAZ in Newcastle took up both the inequalities and public involvement agendas in its aim to promote social inclusion by focusing on local communities and groups that experience health inequalities, and improving care by involving groups in service planning and design. With these principles in mind, multiple complex strategies have been implemented to tackle health inequalities.

The HAZ action plan for Newcastle covers a wide range of health and health-related issues, with six specific areas designated as Areas for Special Action (ASAs): three geographical areas of Newcastle and the Disability, Race Equality and Domestic Violence ASAs. The specific strategies of the HAZ in Newcastle can be characterised as follows:

- partnership and interagency working to achieve change at system and service level
- training and advocacy to enable health care professionals to support and implement change
- peer support and advocacy aimed at empowering individuals and communities to take control of health issues affecting them
- structural change to improve health, including maximising benefits and facilitating housing improvement.

The Health Action Zone initiative emerged in the context of growing emphasis on evidence-based practice in medicine and other health fields (Davies and MacDonald, 1998; Perkins et al., 1999; Greenhalgh and Donald, 2000). Therefore evaluation of the Health Action Zone strategies was considered crucial (Tyne and Wear HAZ, 1999). The aims, strategies and outcomes of complex initiatives, however, produce significant methodological challenges for evaluation (McQueen and Anderson, 2001). Moreover, in the context of a programme that is itself working from principles aimed at empowering communities and alleviating health inequalities, evaluation needed to be conducted in like fashion – collaboratively and integrated in such a way as to contribute to the aims of the projects, not merely as a monitoring function, an add-on or an additional chore.

Evaluation methods

Given the broad range of approaches used within health promotion it is this work, and the developing literature on the evaluation of health promotion, that was turned to in developing strategies for evaluating the diverse projects within the HAZ in Newcastle.[1]

Thorogood and Coombe (2000) describe succinctly the challenges of evaluating health promotion:

> The range of activities involved in health promotion, and the multiple levels of operation, generate difficulties for its evaluation. Each type of activity demands a different form of evaluation. The issue in health promotion evaluation is the accuracy and appropriateness of measurement. This applies equally to quantitative and qualitative study designs. There cannot be just one method for the evaluation of health promotion because the initiatives themselves draw on a variety of methods and disciplines.
>
> pp. 7–8

---

[1] In the Newcastle HAZ a research associate (MJM) was employed within the University of Newcastle to design and coordinate the evaluation of HAZ projects within that division. Evaluation of the Tyne and Wear Health Action Zone was conducted by the University of Northumbria.

Three issues were raised therefore in designing the evaluation of the HAZ in Newcastle: (1) against what measures (outcomes) would it be appropriate to evaluate, (2) what methods would these measures imply and (3) what methodological approach or framework could meet the needs of the projects and the complexity of the endeavour. Each of these is discussed below.

Health outcomes

If we take seriously the claim that understandings and experiences of health are complex, multiple and diverse, and that heterogeneous strategies are necessary for tackling health inequalities, we need therefore to take account of multiple health outcomes in evaluation. In traditional forms of outcome evaluation, health outcomes are viewed in terms of morbidity and mortality. While these outcomes are important, they do not sufficiently describe the range of impacts on health brought about by health promotion initiatives. Thorogood and Coombe (2000) identify the difficulties of evaluating health promotion, in particular the temptation to measure easily quantifiable outcomes (mortality and morbidity) at the risk of ignoring or undervaluing less easily measured effects of health promotion.

In response to this conundrum some writers argue for the measurement of intermediate health outcomes in health promotion (cf. Nutbeam, 1998). In contrast Hepworth (1997) argues for the recognition of the range of effects of health promotion which may themselves be regarded as health outcomes. Hepworth categorises these (p. 236) as health development outcomes (structural determinants, such as transport, food, housing and income), social health outcomes (social factors, such as community and psychological processes, empowerment, participation in decision making, and social and behavioural risk) and biomedical health outcomes (biological factors, such as disease mortality and morbidity). It is in relation to these outcomes that the initiatives of the HAZ in Newcastle were evaluated.

Methods

Given the diversity of the 16 projects of the HAZ in Newcastle, the guiding principles adopted in choosing methods of study were those of appropriateness and rigour advocated by authors, such as Thorogood and Coombe (2000) and Springett (2001), writing about health promotion evaluation. To achieve this the research methods employed to evaluate each project were chosen for their capacity to answer the research question posed in light of the strategies used and the health outcomes envisaged. Health outcomes in the projects in the HAZ in Newcastle were predominantly in the health development (e.g. benefit maximisation, health service training in domestic violence) and social health outcomes (e.g. youth-led peer support, support and advocacy work for families of drug users); some strategies straddled both health development and social health outcomes (e.g. partnership working in the Race Equality ASA).

Research methods included qualitative interview and focus group studies, ethnography, mapping, qualitative and quantitative questionnaires, and statistical analysis of project outputs. The evaluation attended to the intervention and setting, the people, the project and the outcomes. This approach was used not only because it was deemed the most appropriate, but also because attention to the local and specific aspects of the projects would produce the most effective evaluation.

A fundamental principle of the range of strategies employed in the HAZ in Newcastle was a commitment to empowerment and community involvement. It was important, therefore, to respect and maintain this principle in the conduct of the evaluation. In addition the evaluation needed to be useful to the projects, and so a pragmatic and practicable approach was taken. The evaluation had to meet bureaucratic needs – accountability and reporting requirements –and also had to be an integral part of strategies to improve health and change practice. To enhance its utility the evaluation therefore employed a reflexive and iterative process that incorporated feedback and action within the methodology.

Framework

In meeting these requirements the evaluation adopted a set of five key principles. It aimed to:

- employ research design that was methodologically appropriate and systematic
- use multiple methods across a range of research traditions
- be an integral part of strategies to improve health and change practice
- remain supportive and respectful of project values while retaining a critical stance
- work in a collaborative and ethical way, recognising the expertise of participants, workers and researchers.

In accordance with these principles, the most appropriate framework was that of participatory evaluation, which Springett (2001) describes as an approach that 'attempts to involve all who have a stake in the outcome in order to take action and effect change' (p. 83). Chirico et al. (1998) describe the links between participatory evaluation and participatory action research in the context of sustainable community development:

> Participatory Evaluation is a model of evaluation that involves all stakeholders in the project or programme. It draws on 'Participatory Action Research Methodology' which: integrates action, change and research; facilitates learning; ensures that all stakeholders are involved in key decisions, including what to evaluate and how to measure it; encourages empowerment; increases the knowledge base; creates the conditions which ensure the results of the evaluation are acted on and increases relevance.
>
> p. 10

Derived from the participatory action research paradigm, the framework used for the evaluation in the HAZ in Newcastle used a research cycle that included action, evaluation–reflection and development. This model of participatory action evaluation aimed to:

- involve stakeholders in key decisions, including what to evaluate and how to measure it
- integrate action, change and research to ensure the results of the evaluation are acted upon, and thereby increase the relevance
- build capacity in communities and services by facilitating learning, increasing the knowledge base and encouraging empowerment.

Findings, and lessons learnt

To elaborate on the use of the framework and to describe the lessons learnt from its deployment in this setting, the successes of a participatory approach to evaluation are discussed in relation to one of the projects in the HAZ in Newcastle, the Disability ASA. In order to maintain confidentiality, the challenges of participatory evaluation are discussed in relation to all projects, but no project in particular is identified.

Successes

The Disability Area of Special Action project seeks to address inequalities which disabled people experience when accessing mainstream services. The key themes for the work are access and awareness, and the aims, working in partnership with service users and statutory, voluntary and private agencies to improve the health of disabled people, are to:

- influence the development of disability policies, quality standards and development plans, within trusts and services, which reflect good practice
- support the introduction of systems and protocols to promote equality of access

- improve physical access to services through the development of an audit tool for health premises and provision of advice.

An inter-agency implementation group – including a wide range of disability groups and organisations working in related areas, chaired by a disability activist who herself lives with physical disability – oversees the work to implement training with health care personnel, and audits of the accessibility of general practice and other health care premises. The work precedes the introduction of the provisions of the Disability Discrimination Act to ensure accessibility for all people with a physical or learning disability.

The work of the Disability Area of Special Action began with a public conference –involving people with disabilities; statutory, private and voluntary sector organisations; and others interested or involved with disability issues – to discuss and debate the needs of people with disabilities. The inter-agency group was drawn from the participants of this conference, and the report of the conference provided a backdrop for the work and evaluation of the project.

The health outcomes of the project are predominantly health development ones, as the project is directed towards change at the system level: policy, training and upgrading of health care premises. Evaluation was developed with the inter-agency implementation group, and with workers who delivered training and conducted audits. According to the needs of the project the evaluation took three forms:

- a qualitative and quantitative questionnaire on the impact of the audits of health care premises, examining the actions taken by these premises to remedy the impediments to access for people with a disability
- a qualitative questionnaire exploring the appropriateness and usefulness of the training from the perspective of those participating in training sessions
- a qualitative questionnaire clarifying the current and potential role of the interagency group, as it was looking to enhance its role as a catalyst to policy and practice change across primary, secondary and tertiary care facilities in the city.

The project had a limited budget for evaluation and used this to employ two new graduates to conduct the training and audit questionnaires under the supervision of the HAZ research associate (MJM) and the Disability ASA coordinator. The questionnaire to the inter-agency group was administered by the project coordinator. Analysis of all questionnaires and the writing of the evaluation report were conducted jointly by the two research assistants, the project coordinator, an inter-agency group member and the HAZ research associate. Two meetings with the inter-agency group were held to discuss the evaluation and its findings during the analysis and report-writing stages. When the report was nearing completion, a workshop facilitated by the research associate was held in order to develop the recommendations of the evaluation, and to begin to develop an action plan to integrate the findings of the evaluation into the strategic planning processes of the project.

A range of positive outcomes were evident as a result of the evaluation. Collaboration and communication in the process meant that the evaluation met the needs of the project. The work of the Disability ASA was in its infancy: evaluation enabled the inter-agency steering group and the workers to improve their existing work, and to develop work in gaps identified during the evaluation process by the research and by their reflection on that research. The participatory approach to evaluation contributed to the development of projects by actively engaging the project stakeholders in processes to promote clarity, and therefore enable refinement and development of their practice. In this and other projects evaluation became the basis for strategic planning.

Changes in policy meant programmes with a prospective life of several years were curtailed, and the imperative of finding funding to maintain their programmes took on a primary focus in the evaluation. With an emphasis on developing an evidence base and the imperative to mainstream successful projects within a much shorter time frame than originally envisaged, evaluation became an essential tool in succession strategies. Using the evaluation as evidence of the effects of the project, and with their reflection through the process of the evaluation, the Disability ASA team was able to develop innovative strategies for mainstreaming its work. Evaluation in this and other projects was used to demonstrate the importance of the projects, and therefore to establish an argument for their continuation.

Collaboration in evaluation builds capacity. The participatory evaluation process contributes to the development of a research and practice culture that encourages evidence-based practice, as well as developing research skills in individuals. In the Disability ASA the project coordinator developed sufficient confidence to put in place a plan for ongoing evaluation. In other projects community members, project workers and policy makers alike have benefited from the development of research skills, understandings and expertise, and the development of broader understandings of evidence and research.

Challenges

A number of potential problems emerged in the use of participatory forms of evaluation. Three issues in particular require further consideration. The first relates to power relationships in the research setting. It is tempting to assume that the strategy of collaboration in research will disrupt traditional positions in the researcher–researched relationship, and thereby address issues of power. Collaborative approaches may contribute to a renegotiation of this relationship; however, the interaction is a complex one. Structural constraints, for example, that require academic researchers to pursue authorship of publications may conflict with increasingly politicised communities and workers that claim ownership of knowledge. A commitment to participatory and transformative practice in research does not in and of itself ameliorate the problems of power associated with traditional research paradigms; power relations are part of all relationships and therefore require explicit examination. Participatory action evaluation is a step beyond the researcher–subject paradigm, but the relationship between researcher and research participants in collaborative research or evaluation is under-theorised.

Second, there may be contradictions between the principles of participatory evaluation and the evaluation context, particularly where the research is mandatory. Community development approaches, which inform participatory evaluation, advocate working from the agenda of the community. Evaluation is not often drawn from the agenda of the community or group of project workers, and evaluation that is imposed by funders has the potential therefore to change the relationship between evaluator and project stakeholders. Nevertheless, carefully negotiated, participatory approaches offer the potential for evaluation to be a part of the process of change, and not merely to describe or assess it.

Third, participants' expectations of research need to be considered and mutual understandings clarified in order to advance the lessons of evaluation. Stakeholders entered the evaluation process with a range of assumptions and expectations about research. Most often these were drawn from a positivist framework. This was particularly marked for policy makers and project workers with training in biomedical or allied fields. It was necessary, and stimulating, to engage in a dialogue with what could be termed 'lay positivism' in order to broaden understandings about what counts as appropriate methodology. With expectations about the form of research came expectations about the time frame. Projects and their funders do not necessarily work to the same time frame as research. Whether the data collection, analysis and report writing are carried out with or by stakeholders or separately from them, these processes are time-consuming. Yet to be relevant to project development and planning, evaluation needs to be timely.

Moreover, a number of practical considerations need to be taken into account when engaging in collaborative approaches to evaluation: participatory evaluation is resource-intensive. In projects in the HAZ in Newcastle a range of innovative ways were found to resource the evaluation research. In some cases, where it was not appropriate for workers or community members to collect data, postgraduate students and public health trainees took up some of the work as part of their course or training requirements. While this worked to the benefit of all, it is not a sufficient long-term solution. Evaluation needs to be adequately resourced to be effective.

Conclusions and implications for practice

Where due consideration is paid to the issues of power described above, participatory forms of evaluation clearly have advantages for projects and for the communities they work with. Involving all stakeholders in the process of evaluation can enhance the relevance of the work, facilitate the application and integration of evaluation findings and contribute to the processes of change in organisations. Moreover, collaboration in evaluation can build capacity in communities and among workers, thereby contributing to a shift towards evidence-based practice. The use of a range of methodologies in a rigorous and systematic fashion expands among stakeholders, policy makers, workers and community the conceptions of what constitutes evidence.

Acknowledgement

The evaluation of the HAZ in Newcastle involved the collaboration of a range of organisations and individuals. Many thanks are owed to all those who collaborated in the evaluation but particularly to Martin White, Senior Lecturer in the Department of Epidemiology and Public Health, who led the project within the university; Helen Bell, HAZ Coordinator; and Peter Kenrick, Eugene Milne and the members of the Multi-Agency Health Officers Group, whose support was invaluable.

References

Benzeval, M., Judge, K. and Whitehead, M. (1995) *Tackling inequalities in health: an agenda for action*, London: King's Fund.

Black, D., Townsend, P., Davidson, N. and Whitehead, M. (1992) *Inequalities in health: the Black report*, London: Penguin Books.

Bunton, R. and Burrows, R. (1994) *Interventions to promote health in economically deprived areas: a critical review of the literature*, Newcastle upon Tyne: Northern Regional Health Authority, 50.

Chirico, S., Findlay, G., Haywood, L., et al. (1998) *Sustainable community development guidelines*, Luton: Bedfordshire Health Promotion Agency.

Davies, J. K. and MacDonald, G. (eds) (1998) *Quality, evidence and effectiveness in health promotion: striving for certainties*, London: Routledge.

Greenhalgh, T. and Donald, A. (2000) *Evidence based health care workbook: understanding research: for individual and group learning*, London: BMJ.

Hepworth, J. (1997) 'Evaluation in health outcomes research: linking theories, methodologies and practice in health promotion', *Health Promotion International*, 12, 239–50.

McQueen, D. V. and Anderson, L. M. (2001) 'What counts as evidence: issues and debates', in Rootman, I., Goodstadt, M., Hyndman, B., McQueen, D. V., Potvin, L., Springett, J. and Ziglio, E. (eds), *Evaluation in health promotion: principles and perspectives*, WHO Regional Publications, European Series, 92, Copenhagen: World Health Organization.

Nutbeam, D. (1998) 'Health promotion glossary', *Health Promotion International*, 13, 349–64.

Perkins, E. R., Simnett, I. and Wright, L. (eds) (1999) *Evidence-based health promotion*, Chichester: John Wiley.

Springett, J. (2001) 'Participatory approaches to evaluation in health promotion', in Rootman, I., Goodstadt, M., Hyndman, B., McQueen, D. V., Potvin, L., Springett, J. and Ziglio, E. (eds), Evaluation in health promotion: principles and perspectives, WHO Regional Publications, European Series, 92, Copenhagen: World Health Organization.

Thorogood, M. and Coombe, Y. (2000) *Evaluating health promotion: practice and methods*, Oxford: Oxford University Press.

Tyne and Wear HAZ (1999) *A fair chance in life action plan: tackling health inequalities in Tyne and Wear* [available at http://www.haz.co.uk/content/fairchance/actplan.html].

CHAPTER 14

Social capital, health and economy in South Yorkshire coalfield communities

Brigid Kane

The South Yorkshire Coalfields Health Action Zone aims to improve health and reduce health inequalities, and the coalfields' Single Regeneration Budget programme (SRB5) aims to increase labour market participation and rebuild sustainable communities. This research study was commissioned to provide a baseline for future evaluation of both programmes and to demonstrate the linkages between improvements in levels of social capital, health and economic participation.

The issue

The SYC HAZ programme was established on the basis that improving health is not just a question of reducing the incidence of illness and premature mortality, but of improving individuals' and communities' wellbeing and quality of life. This requires action to tackle the wider determinants of health, which include family and social networks, safety and security, educational and economic status, housing, transport and environmental factors.

The HAZ recognised that in order to measure its overall success in the short to medium term a method of measuring changes in wellbeing and quality of life was needed, in addition to outcome and output measures from its activities and standard indicators of morbidity and mortality. At the same time the SRB5 programme was seeking a baseline from which to measure the success of its community capacity building programme in creating sustainable communities and increasing labour market participation.

The HAZ brought together a management group from the two programmes to explore the potential for a joint baseline evaluation study. Over a period of several months the group identified the concept of social capital as underpinning their joint objectives, and reviewed development work being carried out by the

Health Education Authority (now the Health Development Agency) on the links between social capital and health – the Nottingham Social Action Research Project.

A joint SYC HAZ/SRB5 baseline study was agreed, with the following objectives:

- to establish social capital baselines in order to measure change over time
- to investigate links between levels of social capital, labour market measures and self-reported health status
- to make comparisons with national benchmarks
- to provide new evidence to help partners test whether their approach of building community capacity and tackling the wider determinants of health is likely to result in the expected outcomes.

Background

Until relatively recently the economies of the three boroughs of Barnsley, Doncaster and Rotherham were dominated by coal mining. In 1981 there were 39 working pits in the South Yorkshire Coalfields – by 2000, there were just four. The collapse of the coal mining industry has made the South Yorkshire sub-region one of the poorest in the European Union, a fact recognised by its obtaining Objective One status for European structural funding in 2000. In addition to its economic effects and a resultant rise in poverty and ill health, the loss of the 'common bond' of coal mining has had significant negative effects on social cohesion and 'community spirit'.

Focus groups held in four of the study areas held very similar views on community spirit:

- It used to be related to working class identity (manual workers in industries such as mining, steel, textiles, glass). The discipline of the mining industry helped socialise workers, and this regard for other people spilled over into community life.
- It was supported by trade unions, working men's clubs, social and sports clubs, dances and events, neighbourhood pubs. There used to be plenty of leisure-time activities, both political and nonpolitical, offering possibilities for gathering and socialising.
- The big change started in the late 1980s when the mines closed. Mass unemployment started migration into and out of the communities. Closing the mines also affected other businesses in the area.
- Work-related leisure-time activities partly collapsed. Also, private enterprise diminished because of the economic situation (cinemas and shops closed; fewer facilities to provide meeting places).

- Second-generation unemployment has changed family structures and daily routines. Children and young people are lacking social skills and have low aspirations: the economic situation in the communities does not give hope for the future.
- Unemployment is not the only reason for the lack of community spirit. People have more individualistic attitudes, regardless of their social or economic status.
- Residents who have lived in the area for ten years or more are more likely to show interest in community development. This applies also to older generations with personal experience of the coalfields community spirit.
- Respect for public and private property has declined. Graffiti, garbage and vandalism are symptomatic of the decline.
- New initiatives by the communities and by the authorities are helping to foster community spirit, but progress is slow and there are never enough resources to rebuild the areas to the same economic and social levels as before.

Early attempts to regenerate the local economy focused on land reclamation, infrastructure development and business support measures. Current programmes recognise the importance of additional measures to tackle wider social regeneration – seeking to improve educational attainment; retrain the workforce; improve health, housing and the environment; reduce crime and develop sustainable communities.

There are significant 'spillover' effects between these measures. For instance, increasing the skills of residents may enable them to obtain employment: however, if the neighbourhood has not been improved in other ways, they will then move and take their skills and spending power elsewhere. Emigration leads to void houses, and lower incomes to disinvestment in housing repair and maintenance, and to neglect of the immediate environment. As a result there is an increase in the sense of the area's being in decline and in fears about safety, and a reduction in social interaction, as people stay at home more. In addition, if housing quality deteriorates and people become more fearful and isolated, this has a damaging effect on health, which can exacerbate the difficulty of returning to the labour market and contribute to a downward spiral of poverty and poor health.

Approach

The management group selected nine communities to survey: three from each borough. These reflected a balance between pit villages, where prior to 1981 over 25% of working males were employed in mining, inner urban areas and mixed communities. The map in Figure 14.1 shows the nine communities in relation

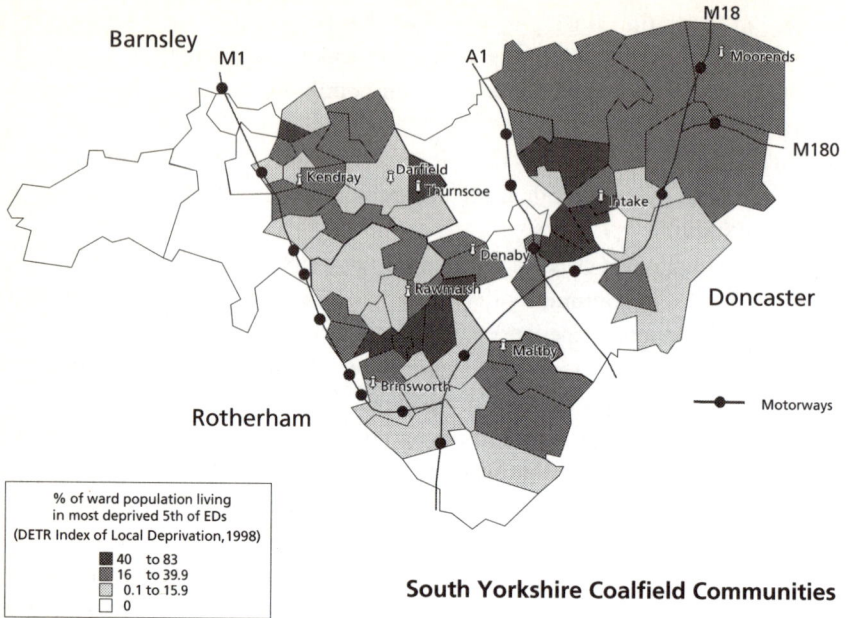

Figure 14.1: Deprivation map

to the percentage of the ward population living in the most deprived fifth of enumeration districts.

The management group and the research team jointly designed the questionnaire, based on a core set of questions derived from the social capital module piloted by the Office of National Statistics (ONS) for the next General Household Survey, supplemented by questions from the HEA's Nottingham Social Action Research Project and a local community study being carried out simultaneously by Sheffield Hallam University. Following consultation with the nine communities, the questionnaire was shortened and adapted, and some community-specific questions were added. The final questionnaire had nine dimensions, as shown in Table 14.1.

The management group, in accordance with the principles of both programmes, decided that the survey should be carried out by residents of the nine communities, with training and support provided by the research team. A total of 52 local people were successfully recruited – through contacts with community workers and local advertising – and trained. They were paid a reasonable rate and travelling expenses, and gained a recognised qualification. A number of them have gone on to full-time education or employment in this field. John and Valerie Grant were not working when they saw the advertisement for interviewers.

Table 14.1 Dimensions of questionnaire

Section	Questions	Section	Questions
Demographics	Address Date of birth Sex Structure of household	Trust and security	System and personal trust Safe at home at night Safe out at night Victim of crime
Neighbourhood	Tenure How long lived in area Satisfaction with area Change in area Satisfaction with facilities Problems with drugs/ alcohol Problems with hooliganism Future	Civic engagement and efficacy	Informed about affairs Involved in local organisation Voting Personal efficacy Working together/influence
		Health	Limiting long-term illness State of health Mental wellbeing Stress
Networks	Neighbourhood networks Contact neighbours/friends, etc.	Lifestyle	Tobacco Fruit and vegetables Healthy diet
Reciprocal help and support	Kind of neighbourhood Favour for a neighbour Help with a lift	Economic	Economic status Training Barriers to employment Skills and qualifications

Equipped by the training course run by Northern College, they surveyed resident opinion in three local communities. John said that the experience was 'stimulating, enjoyable and sometimes very sad. It had a profound effect on both of us'. Both are now working full time with an international market research company. Another interviewer, Lesley Mathieson, used the study as an opportunity to return to work after a break to look after her baby – she has since been on a psychology training course and has started a new administration job with a training company.

The sampling frame was all the residential addresses within the agreed boundaries. A fraction of the properties was selected randomly to give an average of 1350 in each area, with an expected response rate of 33%, to give 450 interviews per area, with a total target of 4000. The response rate was expected to be lower than average as a result of using inexperienced interviewers and a tight timescale. A total of 4217 face-to-face interviews were completed from an amended (to allow for vacant, demolished or difficult to access properties) sample of 9159 properties in the nine communities.

Outcomes and lessons learnt

The survey produced a wealth of data, and multivariate statistical methods were used to model area effects and identify significant associations between aspects of health, the labour market and dimensions of social capital. This enabled the researchers to adjust for age and gender variables in the sample, and to differentiate between the contextual effect of an area and the compositional characteristics of its population: in other words, to determine whether the results were due to the particular group of individuals resident in each community, or whether, as turned out to be the case, some of the results were due to the nature of the place, rather than just the individuals who live in it.

A full report was produced for the partner agencies, and a more user-friendly summary for distribution in the nine communities.[1] Figures 14.2 to 14.8 give some examples of:

- comparisons with national benchmarks
- odds ratios, showing relative levels of indicators across the nine communities
- indexes, showing levels of a social capital factor, such as trust, in each community, constructed using results from a combination of questions
- linkages, showing relationships between elements surveyed – social capital, health, economic and educational status.

Comparison with national benchmarks

Comparisons were made with a number of national benchmarks, where they existed at the time of the survey (more will be possible following the ONS Household Survey, which will include some social capital questions). For example, the residents of the nine coalfields communities were significantly more likely than the national average to be fearful of crime, as shown in Figure 14.2.

Odds ratios

Odds ratios enabled comparisons to be made between the nine communities, and showed a remarkable level of consistency across the communities on factors such as self-reported health indicators, and on levels of social capital measures such as residents' sense of involvement in, and control of, community affairs – so, for example, all aspects of health were generally worse in Kendray and better in Brinsworth. See Figure 14.3.

---

[1] Copies of the report (price £10.00, ISBN 0863399185) are available from: Centre for Regional Economic and Social Research, Sheffield Hallam University, Unit 10, Science Park, Howard Street, Sheffield S1 2LX; tel.: 0114 225 3073; fax: 0114 225 2197. Copies of the summary brochure are available from: South Yorkshire Coalfields Health Action Zone, White Rose House, Ten Pound Walk, Doncaster DN4 5DJ; tel.: 01302 320111; fax: 01302 730613.

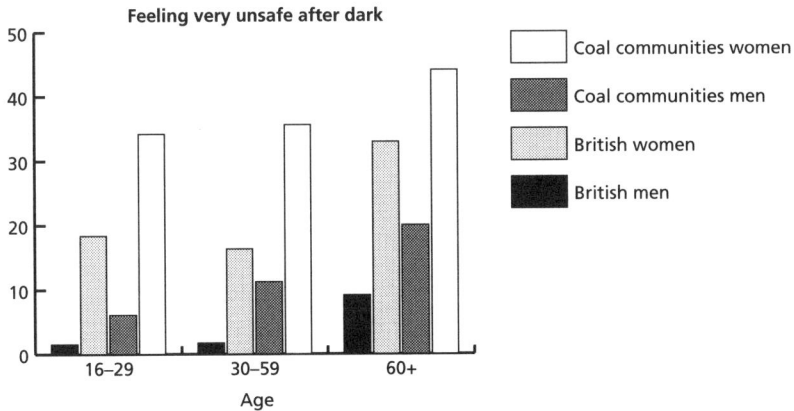

Figure 14.2: Fear of crime

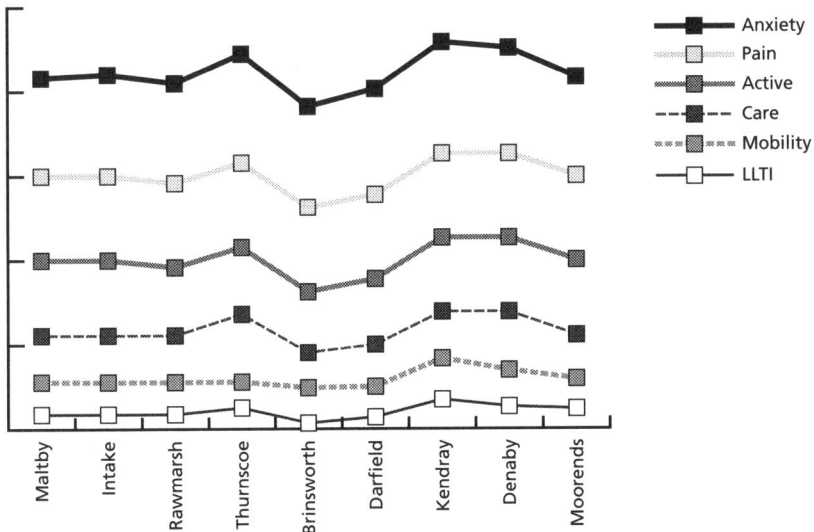

Figure 14.3: Odds ratios: health

Indexes

The combination of questions on indices – of, for example, empowerment and trust – is another way of showing differences between the nine communities. So, for example, people in Moorends are most likely to feel that 'by working together, people in my neighbourhood can influence decisions which affect the neighbourhood' (see Figure 14.4), and people in Intake and Kendray have less

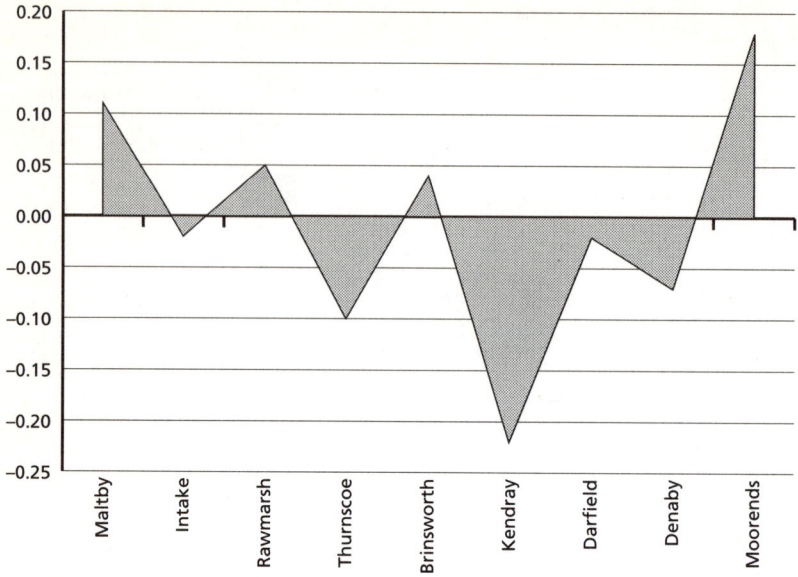

Figure 14.4: Empowerment index

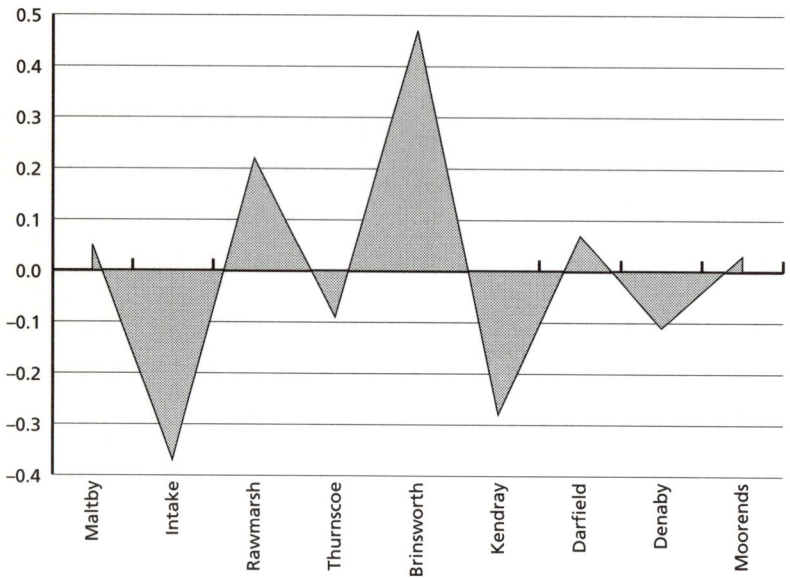

Figure 14.5: Trust index

trust – in family, friends and local politicians – than those in Brinsworth (see Figure 14.5).

Linkages

Analysis of the linkages between factors showed significant relationships. For example, respondents were asked to show their current state of health on a 'thermometer' – those who felt they could ask neighbours for help, or that they were safe at home at night (see Figure 14.6), or had higher qualifications (see Figure 14.7), showed significantly higher levels of health. More than 70% of those with the highest-level qualifications were employed, compared to less than 30% of those without qualifications – see Figure 14.8.

Implications for policy and practice

The SYC HAZ and SRB5 programmes focus on the wider community and encourage the development of neighbourhood networks, trust and participation in community life. All these are elements of social capital, and this report

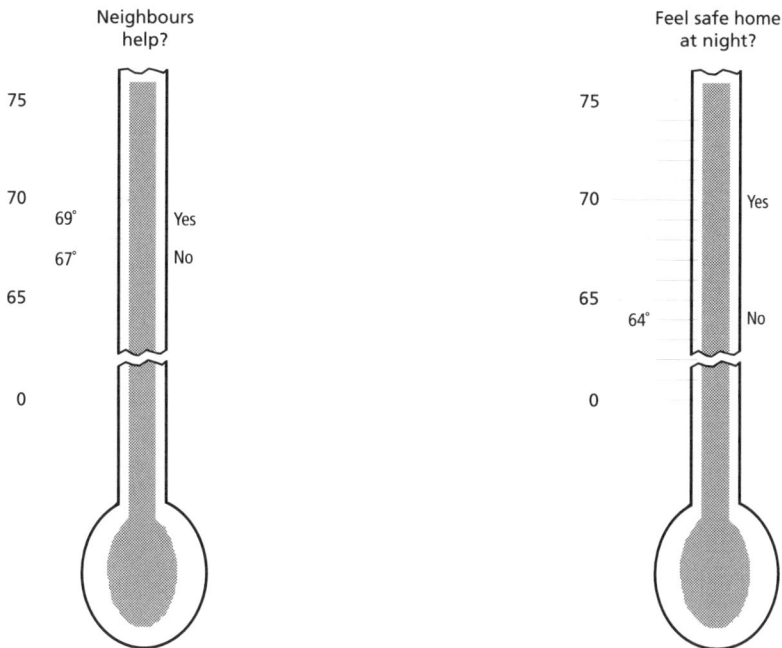

Figure 14.6: Health and reciprocity/health and fear of crime

Better health:
better qualifications

```
80
        78° ──── Highest qualifications
        76° ──── Some qualifications

70
        69° ──── No qualifications

60

 0
```

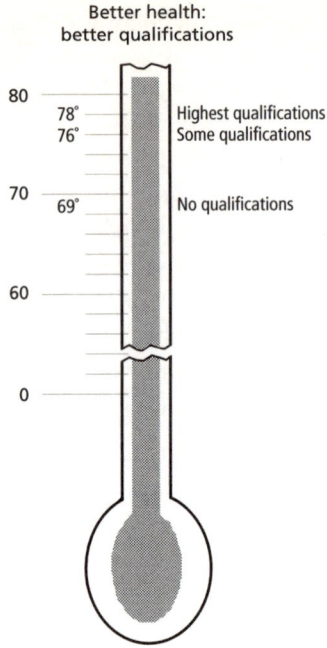

Figure 14.7: Health and qualifications

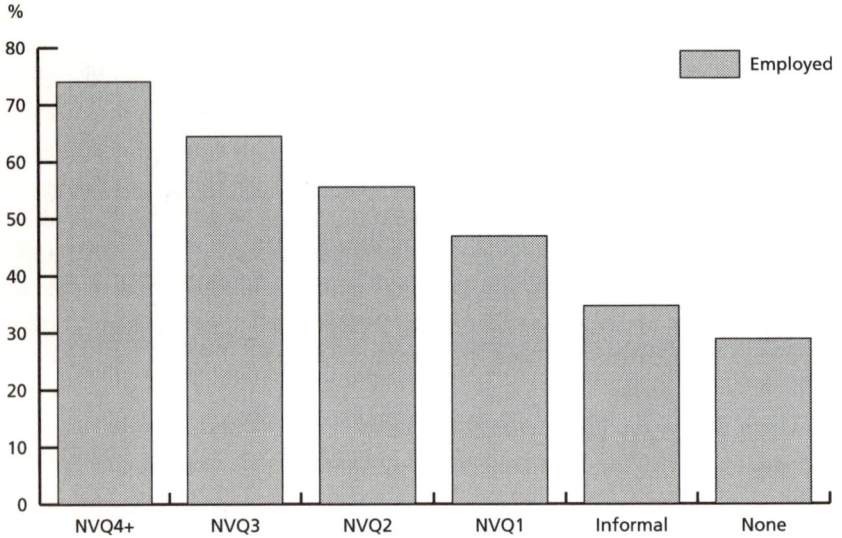

%

```
80 ┐
70 │
60 │
50 │
40 │
30 │
20 │
10 │
 0 └────────────────────────────────────────────
    NVQ4+   NVQ3   NVQ2   NVQ1   Informal   None
```

Employed

Figure 14.8: Qualifications and work

provides ample evidence that higher levels of social capital are linked with better health. This holds both at an individual and community level. If the aims and objectives of the two programmes are met, levels of social capital are therefore expected to increase across the targeted communities. In turn, it is likely that these rising levels of social capital will be associated with improving levels of health and labour market participation.

Like health, social capital is an end in itself – the hallmark of good community life. It is also an integral element of sustainable development both at a community and regional level. Social capital is essential for economic growth and human development. In fact, the World Bank (Grootaert, 1998) has identified four capitals essential to sustainable regeneration. These are:

- fixed capital – buildings, plant, machinery
- environmental capital – natural assets such as minerals and water, which can be enjoyed or exploited
- human capital – a person's 'fitness for work', traditionally defined in terms of skills and qualifications but also, in the light of this research, including health
- social capital – identified by the World Bank as the previously 'missing link', the 'glue' which holds the other capitals together in the development process.

In order to regenerate the coalfields communities and the South Yorkshire region as a whole, it is necessary to have a balanced investment programme in all four capitals.

The SYC HAZ and SRB5 programmes contribute to restoring this balance by investing in the community side of the equation – in both human and social capital. In terms of human capital, the HAZ programme addresses health, especially the issue of disability, which for the men in this survey runs at 60% above the national average. The results show that men reporting some limitation of their mobility are much less likely to engage in the labour market, falling instead into the category 'economically inactive'. The SRB5 programme addresses the qualification and skills element of human capital. Here, too, the baseline results show there is much to be done in the nine communities surveyed, with attainment levels much lower than the national average – indeed less than half the national average in the critical 25–34 age group. The local results also confirm national evidence that the higher a person's qualification, the more likely they are to be in employment.

The results of the survey give some guidance on practical steps for regenerating the area and creating sustainable communities. For instance, the baseline results confirm that community safety is a big issue, with much more fear of crime in the nine communities than the national average. One solution to these fears is 'target hardening' – more locks, gates and walls. A complementary strategy is to improve levels of social capital, especially trust, because the survey demonstrates that higher levels of trust are associated with lower fears for safety. The ultimate result is better mental health and greater wellbeing.

There are as yet no national benchmarks for social capital, so it is not possible to conclude that the coalfields communities rank higher or lower than the British average. However, a comparison of the nine communities indicates important links between social capital, health and labour market participation.

In economic terms Brinsworth and Darfield are the least deprived of the nine communities studied; they also have the highest levels of health and some of the highest levels of social capital, as measured by trust and knowledge of local affairs. It is not possible at this stage to be absolutely sure which of these elements comes first in a sequence of cause and effect, but the survey results do suggest that improved levels of social capital may lead to better health, and better health leads to higher levels of labour market participation. In practical terms, this means that programmes to promote social inclusion may be just as effective in increasing labour market participation as those aimed at raising the levels of qualifications.

Overall, the study has demonstrated significant links between improvements in social capital, health and economic factors. The complex and mutually reinforcing interactions between these factors are difficult to untangle, but the study does suggest that the holistic approach taken by the SYC HAZ – working in and with communities, alongside support for direct interventions in health and social services, education, housing, training, employment and crime reduction – is likely to produce the intended improvements in health and wellbeing. The planned follow-up study will, it is hoped, provide evidence that the interventions made by the SYC HAZ and SRB5 programmes have made a real difference to people's lives.

Acknowledgement

This paper presents a study carried out on behalf of the SYC HAZ and the South Yorkshire SRB5 Programme 'Helping Communities to Build a Better Future', supported by Yorkshire Forward, the Regional Development Agency. The research was managed by a partnership group, with members from the local and health authorities of Barnsley, Doncaster and Rotherham. The research team consisted of Geoff Green and Ann Suokas, Centre for Regional Economic and Social Research; Mike Grimsley, Computing and Management Sciences; and Rachel Linacre, Survey and Statistical Research Centre (all Sheffield Hallam University); and Margaret Prescott and Tony Jowitt (both Northern College).

Reference

Grootaert, G. (1998) *Social capital: the missing link?*, SCI Working Paper, 3, April, Washington, DC: World Bank.

CHAPTER 15

Learning from theory-driven evaluations across local Health Action Zone initiatives in Nottingham: using or losing?

Dara Coppel

Context

Nottingham Health Action Zone

Nottingham Health Action Zone (HAZ) is a second-wave HAZ, initiated in April 1999, which originally aimed to focus on reducing health inequalities among children and families. The devolvement of funding to 11 workstreams, 6 primary care groups (PCGs), the voluntary sector, 200 projects, 3 HAZ Innovation Initiatives, 6 local HAZ fellowships and a national HAZ fellow made it a highly innovative, complex programme. How to evaluate the local initiatives in a practicable, pragmatic, straightforward manner for researchers and non-researchers alike was immediately raised as an issue. In response, a purpose-designed evaluation resource pack (Coppel, 1999) was disseminated to all projects, alongside the provision of workshops and training to key project stake-holders to ensure that they had the necessary skills to adequately tackle self-evaluation using a social scientific model – namely the theories of change (Connell et al., 1995).

Area-based initiatives (ABIs)

Over the past twenty years, government departments have introduced area-based initiatives to address cumulative social, economic and physical problems in dis-advantaged areas (DETR, 2000). Given the plethora of local area initiatives there still remains a lack of evidence as to the specific impacts that they have achieved. Cynics believe that 'demonstration' projects create a flurry of activity, at low cost, but have little lasting impact (Higgins, 1998). According to a review by the Department of the Environment, Transport and the Regions (DETR, 2000) on the evidence base of regeneration policy and practice, it is the diversity in evaluation approaches and constraints on evaluation practice across area-based regeneration that have limited the degree to which informed and rigorous lessons can be drawn.

According to Higgins (1998) there were higher hopes for HAZs. They were expected to create opportunities to allow achievements to become mainstreamed, with new ways of working to become the norm across England. This chapter attempts to look at how effective Nottingham HAZ has been in maximising the application of learning and new behaviour into core activities of organisations and policies. The discussion specifically explores whether the approach that Nottingham HAZ has taken in providing evidence is useful and acceptable to local service decision-makers and policy makers.

Mechanisms

Evaluation

Public initiatives and programmes like the HAZ are complex social processes, and thus traditional experimental research is deficient. Evaluations such as randomised controlled trials (RCTs) have been criticised for not reflecting 'real world' conditions (Severs, 2000). Patton (1980) argues that research is aimed at 'truth', while evaluation is about the production of information to influence policy making and to improve effectiveness.

There are a wide range of views about what evaluation is, and the term 'evaluation' is often misunderstood. According to Shaw (2000) this has resulted in its being an often abused term in relation to public programmes. Nottingham HAZ therefore attempted to standardise the evaluation methods and terminology used across the HAZ by encouraging the use of the theories of change evaluation framework (Connell et al., 1995), and promote the use of pre-defined terminology as stated within the purposely devised evaluation resource pack (Coppel, 1999).

Theories of change

So why did Nottingham choose to use the theories of change? Theory-driven evaluation is an evaluation method that claims to deal with process rather than just outcomes (Shaw, 2000). Its basic concept is that it is the theories behind a programme, as identified by key stakeholders themselves, that are evaluated. It was Weiss (1972) who was the first to seriously argue for the need to base evaluation on the theories underlying initiatives. Weiss believes that it is the breaking down and demonstration of a series of micro-steps that lead from inputs to outcomes that make the idea of causal attribution more understandable. The evaluation can trace each step along the route to see whether the stages appear as anticipated: 'If things go as expected, the evaluation can tell *how* the programme worked in achieving its goals; it can explain the steps and processes that led to desired results. If data do not confirm some of the steps, the evaluation can show where the programme goes off the tracks' (Weiss, 1998, 59). As Chen and Rossi (1987) state, theory-based evaluation helps to assure that the results identified are firmly connected to what the programme has been doing and that they are a consequence of the programme's activities.

HAZs were created as learning enterprises (Bauld et al., 2000). Luckily a proportion of the HAZ programme expenditure was allocated to evaluation from the outset, which resulted in the setting up of a national HAZ evaluation team. This team strongly encouraged the use of the theories of change evaluation framework at both a national and local level.

Dissemination of evaluation findings

Nottingham HAZ is in the process of disseminating and devolving widely much of what has been learnt from the HAZ over the past three years, which, according to the evidence, is unlike previous ABIs (LGA, 2000). The Local Government Association (ibid.) suggested that the majority of learning from area-based initiatives is usually retained at the centre. The local strategy for dissemination attempts to apply numerous approaches not only to ensure that effective initiatives continue, but to ensure that effective ways of working are incorporated into everyday service delivery. According to Dixon (2000) it is people, rather than electronics, that transfer knowledge, and Dixon therefore emphasises the importance of involving people at all stages of the best-practice identification process and in dissemination.

Uncertainty as to the continuation of the HAZ can only be detrimental in the transferring of learning, as people are moving into new positions to secure employment beyond the proposed life of the HAZ. Given these circumstances which cannot be avoided, Nottingham HAZ has methods in place to ensure that the right parties are engaged in decision making. Frontline workers, workstream leads and strategic players have played a part in sifting through the 200 projects to determine which are worth funding in the future.

Each key organisation across the district was brought together for a 'mainstreaming' day whereby all representatives outlined their key priorities within their own organisations. This was followed by the production of an assessment-criteria grid, which determined to what degree each project hit on each of the different priority areas. In addition, information was sought on how well the projects had included the community, how well the projects had worked in partnership, how well they had built in evaluation and produced evidence, and finally how successful they proved to be. It was this 'grid' process that was then used as a feeding mechanism to the different organisations – such as the city council, local strategic partnership (LSP), health authority leads, primary care trusts, etc. – which it is hoped will enable projects to be picked up by other agencies if deemed useful and beneficial to the population they serve. It is hoped that this process of ensuring that effective initiatives continue will be helped by maximum stakeholder and frontline staff/user involvement.

Ensuring effective ways of working is as important as the continuation of projects as a whole. Nottingham HAZ is currently undertaking a mix of practices in developing, defining and disseminating best working practice. It is hoped that people will be more inclined to adopt or develop good practice if they identify for themselves what will work best in their own circumstances, with the opportunity to learn and discuss. Strategies are currently being written to develop and utilise the learning from the HAZ pertinent to individual organisations' needs. The individual organisations' own structures and processes will affect the embedding of good practice. The HAZ therefore needs to ensure that the preferred mechanism for receiving information is identified across the different organisations, taking into consideration that there may be several different types of knowledge that need to be transferred, each calling for a different transfer method.

According to the Office for Public Management, the more complex the best practice to be shared, the more interactive and 'face to face' the approach needed (OPM, 2000). One local example of an area where there was a wealth of complex learning involved projects that aimed to reach and include black and ethnic minority groups. Ill feeling was evident among some local project workers that the HAZ failed to do enough to tackle health inequalities among black and ethnic minority groups, so, to prevent history repeating itself, Nottingham HAZ has since commissioned some 'whole system' facilitators to bring together key stakeholders to tease out the issues and learning.

The OPM (2000) also recognises that guidance materials are often best used within a wider coordinated dissemination strategy. One such area of knowledge that lends itself to that transfer mechanism is the learning from the local HAZ Fellowship Scheme. Nottingham HAZ, in partnership with Trent Focus (an organisation funded by NHSE Trent to promote the development of research in primary care), has carried out an evaluation of the scheme to identify the extent to which giving frontline staff a chance to carry out research has increased their capacity to undertake evaluation, and influence service delivery. The evaluation findings strongly support the investment in local fellowships and a good practice guide is being written, in partnership, to disseminate across the district. Other guidance material that the HAZ produces includes: bimonthly HAZ newsletters, which are used to bring to people's attention progress and learning from the HAZ, and the production of a HAZ directory of all HAZ projects and their progress to date. Regularly updated guidance such as these tends to be financially draining and labour-intensive, and it remains unclear as to how well used they are.

Another method of dissemination being used by Nottingham HAZ to encourage the take-up of good working practice is via personal contact and experience. The literature suggests that people like to see/hear about good practice from another person and experience it for themselves (LGA, 2000) – hence Nottingham HAZ's recent HAZ Conference for 400 people, which incorporated keynote speakers, workshops and interactive display sessions. Nottingham stakeholders also frequently speak at seminars and workshops both locally and nationally to share learning.

The OPM (2000) believes that strategies which allow for continuing contact (as opposed to 'one-offs') through networks and other interactive systems are important. Networks certainly have increased in popularity among policy makers. One local network that has created a forum for such discussions is named the 'Subregional Evaluation Network'. This was initiated to provide an opportunity for representatives from ABIs and statutory and voluntary services across the region to discuss evaluation methods, key learning, recommendations and the future of services. Questionnaires distributed (jointly by Nottingham HAZ and Nottingham City Council) across the region have highlighted the demand for such a network. The test will be to make sure that the network does not become cliquish and that it remains as inclusive as is possible. It is hoped that the network will incorporate elements of meeting and sharing of experiences between individuals in a way that encourages a continuing process of feedback on what works well, building on what has been developed by others. The effectiveness of the network remains to be seen, and will undoubtedly depend upon such factors as: levels of involvement, the extent of trust and leadership, and support and commitment from participating organisations.

There is no doubt that Nottingham HAZ, in line with key literature recommendations, offers a variety of approaches within one 'learning' strategy to promote change (NHS Centre for Reviews and Dissemination, 1999). What remains to be seen is how well the evidence and recommendations are utilised.

Outcomes

Utilisation of results in influencing local service decision-making

With a clear dissemination strategy under way within Nottingham HAZ, it would be misleading to believe that this in itself will lead to changes in local services. Unfortunately, for many reasons, the non-use of evaluation findings is all too common (Weiss, 1998).

One explanation as to why evaluation findings may not be taken on board is the common belief that social scientific evaluation methods produce findings that aren't generalisable, and therefore are of limited use to other service decision-makers.

Lack of certainty about the acceptance of the recommendations made from using the theories of change model may prove to be an effective inhibitor of change. According to the DETR, criticisms of ABIs are that most evidence has tended to focus on individual projects with insufficient attention paid to context, which inhibits the transfer of reliable findings and learning across projects (DETR, 2000).

By utilising the theories of change, Nottingham HAZ has gone beyond not only determining whether something works but has attempted to identify *what* has made initiatives work, by taking into consideration the context within which it is based. In addition it has attempted to explore causality between impacts and projects, as well as identify links between project design and outcomes experienced – something recognised to have been lacking in evaluations of previous ABIs (DETR, 2000). It is hoped that the HAZ in Nottingham has been a useful mechanism in helping service decision-makers appreciate social research, as opposed to just seeing the need to draw on medical research and management sciences that produce performance figures in terms of economy, efficiency and effectiveness (Beattie, 1995). A recent research report by the Office for Public Management stated that people need to trust the source of the data if they are to take it on board (OPM, 2000), and Nottingham has certainly made every attempt to encourage this.

According to the DETR, the evidence base with respect to good practice from ABIs often comes too late to influence further schemes and mainstream services (DETR, 2000). Even if decision makers are willing to accept good practice and recommendations, the timing of the 'learning' dissemination is crucial. Primary care trusts are seen to be 'the vanguard of community-based initiatives to narrow the health gap...across the UK' (Marks and Hunter, 2000, 8), and it is essential that they absorb HAZ learning, yet their decision-making processes are taking place six months before the HAZ programme is due to finish. Nottingham HAZ has therefore had to compromise and provide short-term interim learning.

Weiss (1998) believes that one of the reasons that organisations fail to take the lessons of evaluations to heart is that they find the status quo a contentedly feasible state, and that changing practices takes money, a factor often in short supply. This is clearly not the case for the recently formed primary care trusts (PCTs), which are currently undergoing changes of practices and habits of staff within many local structures – surely, then, this is a crucial time for HAZ to intercept? However, not surprisingly, fairly embryonic organisations such as PCTs and LSPs will be more concerned with survival and meeting inflicted national targets and criteria. It must be remembered that even with good evidence, all organisations have restricted funding, service specific targets and have other inflexibilities (LGA, 2000). Nottingham HAZ needs to portray the learning in terms of a change of ways of working that doesn't need huge financial backing. Luckily both the local PCTs and LSP have a culture which is supportive of knowledge management and transfer, but the HAZ cannot afford to become complacent, and needs to continually ensure that this remains the case.

Utilisation of results in influencing policy

Alongside trying to discover whether the HAZ programme or its individual initiatives work, and why, there is an obvious role for evaluation to play in influencing government policy-making. A current debate examines whether social scientists can adequately address even the most basic questions being asked, such as whether policies work and how cost effective the interventions are (Walker, 2001). It is frustrating that policy makers have not awaited the results of the impact evaluations of HAZ before they have taken decisions on implementing more initiatives such as local strategic partnerships. The eagerness of politicians to see change could potentially see the same wheels reinvented and history repeating itself once again. The HAZ will not be able to change the way in which policy systems work. It can, however, attempt to influence the development of new government structures using the vast amount of knowledge that has been accumulated over the past the years. Nottingham HAZ, similar to all HAZs across England, cannot afford to sit on the results, citing the difficulties of the initiative and its evaluation, the inadequacy of its resources, the changing of the priorities and the possible shortening of the HAZ life. According to Craig (2000), the growing pressure from government to engage in evaluation has permeated local government, the health service and the voluntary sector, through pressures to demonstrate identifiable outputs and the emphasis on the right of consumers to receive quality services of defined standards.

It is therefore hoped that the policy makers will be more receptive to the implications of all HAZ interim evaluation results. At a minimum, Nottingham HAZ, alongside other HAZ evaluations and the national evaluation, will have at least made a contribution in raising new issues and altering the nature and climate of discussions.

Conclusion

It certainly isn't clear as to whether any of the previous good practice from area-based initiatives has been retained from 30 years ago (LGA, 1999). While Nottingham HAZ has most definitely encouraged creative initiatives at the local level, the impact it has had on reducing health inequalities across the district is uncertain. Nottingham HAZ and its use of the theories of change cannot claim to be able to answer all questions, yet there is no doubt that it has played a very valuable role in influencing services locally, an extremely challenging task. It is high time the government accepted the need for long-term views on designing and delivering programmes, as well as long-term views on constructing and disseminating an appropriate evidence base. However, whether or not the HAZ receives more funding from the Department of Health, it is hoped that the good practice that is currently being built into longer-term planning and investment in strategic frameworks across the district will endure.

References

Bauld, L., Judge, K., Lawson, L., Mackenzie, M., Mackinnon, J. and Truman, J. (2001) *Health Action Zones in transition: progress in 2000*, Glasgow: University of Glasgow.

Beattie, A. (1995) 'Evaluation in community development for health: an opportunity for dialogue', *Health Education Journal*, 54, 465–72.

Chen, H. and Rossi, P. (1987) 'The theory driven approach to validity', *Evaluation and Programme Planning*, 10, 95–103.

Connell, J. P., Kubisch, A. C., Schorr, L. B. and Weiss, C. H. (eds) (1995) *New approaches to evaluating community initiatives: concepts, methods and contexts*, Washington, DC: The Aspen Institute.

Coppel, D. (1999) 'An evaluation resource for Nottingham HAZ projects' [unpublished].

Craig, G. (2000) *Evaluation: the social policy perspective*, Research Seminar on Evaluation Research, Nottingham: Trent Focus.

DETR (2000), *A review of the evidence base for regeneration policy and practice*, Regeneration Research Summary 39.

Dixon, N. (2000) *Common knowledge in people management*, Institute of Personnel Development, 17 February.

Higgins, J. (1998) 'HAZs warning', *Health Service Journal*, 16 April, 24–5.

LGA (1999) *Supporting action zones: some early lessons from area-based initiatives*, London: LGA Publications.

LGA (2000) *Supporting the action zones: early messages, future plans*, London: LGA Publications.

Marks, L. and Hunter, D. (2000) *From PCGs to PCTs: work in progress*, Bath, UK: Medical Management Services.

NHS Centre for Reviews and Dissemination (1999) *Effective health care: getting evidence into practice*, University of York, February.

OPM (2000) *The effectiveness of different mechanisms for spreading best practice*, London: Office for Public Management.

Patton, M. Q. (1980) *Qualitative evaluation methods*, Newbury Park: Sage.

Severs, M. (2000) 'Complex service evaluation', *Age and Ageing*, 29-S2, 5–7.

Shaw, I. (2000) *Evaluating public programmes: contexts and issues*, Aldershot: Ashgate Publishing Company.

Walker, R. (2001) 'Great expectations: can social science evaluate New Labour's policies?', *Evaluation*, 7/3, 305–30.

Weiss, C. (1972) *Evaluation research*, New Jersey: Prentice-Hall Inc.

Weiss, C. (1998) *Evaluation*, 2nd edn, New Jersey: Prentice-Hall Inc.

Section 3

Innovation

Michaela Benzeval and Fiona Meth

When Health Action Zones were established they were seen to be central to the government's agenda to reduce health inequalities. This was partly because HAZs themselves were mainly located in disadvantaged areas, and hence additional investment in them was part of the government's strategy to focus on the 'worst off':

> Health Action Zones are a key part of the Government's drive to target areas with particularly high levels of ill health...and so improve the health of the worst off at a faster rate than the general population. This is the first time a British Government has set itself such a task.
>
> Dobson, 1998

However, equally importantly, HAZs were expected to act as 'trailblazers' and to lead the way in developing new ways of tackling local health inequalities: 'Health Action Zones are in the vanguard of our new approach to tackling health inequalities and promoting new ways of working together locally between health and social services' (Denham, 1999); 'Health Action Zones are in the frontline of the Government war on health inequalities. They have both the opportunity and the responsibility to pioneer new ways of driving up local standards of health' (Jowell, 1999).

As pioneers or trailblazers in tackling health inequalities, HAZs had not only to invest in innovative initiatives, but also to establish effective ways of learning from them. They were expected both to mainstream successes internally and to disseminate good practice more broadly to the health community. HAZs were supported in their endeavours with core funding, opportunities to bid for additional innovation grants, and development support from a central DoH unit.

In response to these challenges, HAZs have developed strategies to tackle health inequalities that vary considerably in their goals, content and focus (Benzeval and Meth, 2002). For example, while some HAZs are aiming to reduce inequalities between different parts of their HAZ, others are aiming to increase overall health within their HAZ towards the English average. All HAZs have strategies to address health inequalities, which include:

- tackling the root causes of ill health, such as poor housing, unemployment and low incomes
- promoting community cohesion and empowering people in disadvantaged circumstances
- creating opportunities for healthy lifestyles
- improving access to health services.

Finally, all HAZs are targeting their efforts in order to reduce inequalities. Some HAZs are concentrating on investing in particular disadvantaged geographic areas within their boundaries; others are emphasising the needs of people experiencing socioeconomic disadvantage; some are focusing on the needs of particular groups, such as black and ethnic minorities; while others are prioritising people with particular health problems. Many HAZs also originally placed considerable emphasis on the needs of children, which has more recently been identified as a national priority to address health inequalities (Acheson, 1998; DoH, 2001).

Within these strategies there are numerous specific initiatives. In the first report of the national evaluation of Health Action Zones, we identified over 750 individual projects in the implementation plans of the 26 zones (HAZ National Evaluation Team, 1999). Learning from these projects is vital to the endeavour of HAZs in tacking health inequalities locally and generating useful learning for other areas. Chapters 17 to 21 describe innovative projects from five HAZs that aim to reduce health inequalities for different groups of the population by addressing a range of causal mechanisms within the social pathways to health. As such they are microcosms of the whole HAZ enterprise.

Chapter 16 suggests that innovation in HAZs has been made more difficult by changing national priorities. Using Teesside as a case study it illustrates how local stakeholders responded to the change in priorities with the emergence of the modernisation agenda in 1999. Evidence from the national evaluation more broadly suggests that this did change local priorities considerably (Bauld et al., 2001). Moreover, within the NHS more generally, despite the government's rhetoric, health inequalities have never been seen as a 'first order priority' (Benzeval and Meth, 2001). Nevertheless, there is still a significant amount of innovative work on reducing inequalities. It is on these kinds of investment that we focus here. The following section explores what is being done within the projects described in more detail in subsequent chapters, how they are innovative, and what can be learnt from them at this stage in their efforts to reduce health inequalities effectively.

The initiatives

Table 1 overleaf briefly highlights some of the basic characteristics of the innovative projects described in Chapters 17 to 21. For each project it summarises: the outcomes targeted for improvement, the types of activities the project is engaged in, the groups it is targeting, any problems it has encountered, how the HAZ is involved in the project and any evaluation findings to date. The five projects have many aspects in common.

The main aim of the majority of the projects is to improve the self-esteem and the self-confidence of participants, and as a result to improve their health. The only project which does not have this objective (income maximisation in Camden and Islington, Chapter 18) aims to increase the incomes of the targeted groups. Two of the other projects – the Leicestershire education and training workstream (Chapter 21) and Let's Get Serious (Chapter 17) – also aim to improve income by providing employment to targeted groups. Three of the projects – the Pampering Gang (Chapter 19), Stepping Out (Chapter 20) and Let's Get Serious – are also concerned with improving community cohesion. Only two of the projects have explicit aims that relate to health services. The Leicestershire workstream hope to improve the sensitivity and appropriateness of their services, while it is hoped the groups targeted by the Pampering Gang will make more effective use of services. However, both Stepping Out and the income maximisation project suggest that there have been (welcome) reductions in the use of health services as a consequence of their activities.

To achieve their outcomes the projects are addressing a range of causal mechanisms within social pathways to health. The Camden and Islington project is the most straightforward, by providing benefit advice to increase the incomes of the local population, although it has a range of different outreach and targeting schemes to achieve this. Two of the projects – Let's Get Serious and the Leicestershire initiative – emphasise providing education, training and employment to disadvantaged groups. A number of the projects place emphasis on providing social and emotional support either through the initiative itself, as in Let's Get Serious, or through peer group activities, as in the Pampering Gang and Stepping Out. The primary activities in the last two, however, are focused on lifestyle issues through providing beauty and alternative therapies, and exercise and leisure opportunities. Finally, the education and training initiative in Leicestershire is mainly focused on training the NHS workforce to improve their ability to work with different client groups in order to make services more appropriate and sensitive to their needs. However, in doing this it provides employment opportunities for disadvantaged groups within its community.

All of the projects target their efforts on particular groups that experience health or socioeconomic disadvantage. Stepping Out and the education and training programme in Leicestershire both place considerable emphasis on

Table 1 Basic characteristics of innovative projects

Project (chapter no.)	Outcomes targeted for improvement	Services offered	Groups targeted	Problems encountered	HAZ involvement	Evaluation findings/lessons
Let's Get Serious (17)	Education, employment, emotional support, self-confidence and self-esteem, health and wellbeing, healthy lifestyles, community cohesion	Providing training, employment and support to unemployed men who then act as mentors to provide emotional support to schoolboys	Men who are unemployed and boys at risk of exclusion living in disadvantaged areas	Practical problems within project; problems with interface to mainstream services; negative publicity	National HAZ Innovation Fund	External evaluation to be commissioned; no details provided
Income maximisation in Camden and Islington (18)	Income, on the assumption that it will improve health	Giving benefits advice in primary care settings	People on low incomes	Problems with interface to mainstream services	HAZ provided funding for continuation or expansion of a number of pre-existing projects	Evaluation conducted by HAZ: • For every £10,000 invested, client income can be increased by £100,000. • More appropriate use of services.
Pampering Gang (19)	Social support and networks, self-confidence, self-esteem, health, healthy lifestyles and appropriate use of health services	Providing regular group 'pampering' sessions with crèche facilities	Women living in disadvantaged areas and hence their children	Negative publicity; practical problems within project	Pilot undertaken prior to HAZ: HAZ provided funding for subsequent sessions	To be externally evaluated with respect to women's wellbeing
Stepping Out (20)	Physical activities, social networks, self-esteem of people with disabilities; awareness of their needs among leisure staff; integration into community	Providing exercise and other group leisure activities, plus transport to facilities	People with disabilities	Practical problems within project; problems with interface to mainstream services	Pilot undertaken prior to HAZ: HAZ now funds project	Self-evaluation by project: • Improvements in self-reported health, self-worth, social contacts • Reduced use of mainstream services
Education and training workstream, Leicestershire (21)	Skills, employment, income, self-confidence and self esteem; sensitivity and appropriateness of health care	Providing training, mainly for staff; providing employment; improving recruitment and retention within the NHS	People with mental health problems, BEMGs, asylum seekers and refugees	None discussed	HAZ funds dedicated staff to develop and support initiatives and pilot projects	External evaluation proposed; no details provided

improving the health and circumstances of people with health problems. All of the projects, except Stepping Out, also focus on people who are socially and/or economically disadvantaged: people on low incomes or who are unemployed, those living in deprived areas, and schoolchildren who are at risk of marginalisation. Two of the projects – in Leicestershire and in Camden and Islington – also target the needs of black and ethnic minority groups (BEMGs).

Four of the projects describe some of the problems that they have encountered as they implemented their plans. In the main these are specific practical problems associated with that particular project. For example, difficulties finding accommodation for the Pampering Gang, or problems of working with single-handed GPs in the income maximisation project. In other projects the problems relate to their reliance on mainstream services in some ways. For example, Stepping Out found that public transport was wholly inadequate for their needs and that there were problems with the physical access to some of the leisure services. Let's Get Serious encountered many delays as a result of the checks that needed to be run on potential mentors who would be working with children. Finally, both the Pampering Gang and Let's Get Serious received negative media publicity about their providing 'treats' to 'undeserving people' or giving them roles of trust.

The HAZ is investing resources in all of the projects: in some cases modestly, e.g. £5000 for one year of the Pampering Gang, and in others rather more substantially, e.g. £2 million from the HAZ Innovation Fund over three years for Let's Get Serious. In some cases the HAZ is the sole funder; in others it is one of a number of different sources of funding. In particular, in at least three of the five examples, the projects themselves or pilot schemes had already begun before the HAZ became involved.

Given that HAZs were envisioned as innovative learning organisations, the undertaking of robust evaluation is paramount. Only two project evaluations have been completed so far; however, all the projects do plan to undertake them. Had these been conducted in tandem with the projects' development and implementation, they might have contributed to this process, as well as creating valuable learning for future efforts to address health inequalities.

Of the two projects that have been evaluated – Stepping Out and the income maximisation project in Camden and Islington – evidence suggests that the projects have achieved their aims. More extensive descriptions of the evaluation methods and findings could help in drawing out this evidence further. Neither of these evaluations appears to have adopted a theories of change or logic approach, and more structured thinking on causality would make it easier to identify what particular mechanisms within the projects have contributed to the desired changes (Pawson and Tilley, 1997).

How are the projects innovative?

Most of the chapters in this section point to the key characteristics that they believe make the projects innovative, and are part of the reason for their success and/or are central to what they are trying to achieve. These include:

- being an interagency initiative
- empowering users, individuals and groups
- being multifaceted and holistic
- adopting a social model of health
- targeting groups in particular need
- providing intensive and sensitive tailored support
- using outreach to make contact with 'hard to reach' groups.

Interagency action

All of the projects described are based on collaborations between a range of statutory and private agencies. Such partnerships are vital to the projects as different agencies bring different resources, skills and knowledge to the table. For example, the Pampering Gang relies on local colleges and businesses to provide beauticians, hairdressers and beauty products, a housing association to provide accommodation, and a local childcare organisation to provide a crèche, as well as the health visitors and other health care staff to organise the overall programme. Given the complex needs of many of the groups targeted in these initiatives and the multifaceted response required from services, no single organisation has the capacity or expertise to address all of the needs by itself. Partnership working therefore appears to be an essential underpinning of the kinds of projects described here.

Empowering users and groups

A fundamental principle underlying most of the projects outlined in this section is the need to empower the groups with whom they are working. Some of the projects, for example, Stepping Out and the Pampering Gang, are user-initiated, and have had significant user involvement in designing the initiative. Similarly, many of the specific schemes within the education and training workstream in Leicestershire are designed and led by particular user groups as a way of improving the care they receive. More integrally, a number of the initiatives, most clearly embodied by Let's Get Serious, are actually designed to provide support to individuals to enable them to take more control over their own lives. While it is a direct aim of this initiative, such empowerment is also an underlying feature of many of the others.

Being multifaceted and holistic

Most of the projects are multifaceted, and see this as an important part of their strategy to meet the complex needs of the individuals concerned and to improve the broad outcomes that they wish to achieve. Most argue that they need to adopt a holistic approach to individuals' circumstances in order to improve their health. For example, Stepping Out combines group social activities with physical exercise and transport. Similarly, the Pampering Gang combines social activities with beauty sessions, alternative therapies and childcare. Let's Get Serious aims to help both mentors and mentees, by tackling, among other things, issues of employment, training, education, social support, lifestyles and income. Not all of the projects described are this complex, however. The income maximisation initiative focuses exclusively on increasing the incomes of people on a low income, although it employs a range of delivery models to do so.

Social model of health

Linked to the need to be holistic is the fact that all of the initiatives have an underlying social model of health. They recognise the need to address a range of issues in the complex social pathways that create ill health, in order to improve health and to reduce health inequalities. While a number of the initiatives are based in health care settings or primarily run by health care professionals, they all tackle social and economic determinants of health, such as income, education, employment and training, as well as social support. Only one initiative – the Leicestershire education and training workstream – has a significant emphasis on health care services, but even this initiative has dual goals. So while it focuses on improving the sensitivity and the appropriateness of services, it works with user groups to provide training for staff, creating employment opportunities for users and improving the skills of its workforce.

Targeting

All of the initiatives described in this section invest their efforts in particular groups of the population and in some cases in particular geographic areas. They focus on improving the circumstances and health of the most disadvantaged groups in order to reduce social exclusion and health inequalities. In the main these initiative have targeted people who are socially and economically disadvantaged, but in two cases they focus on people with health problems which themselves cause social and economic exclusion. By focusing efforts on those groups that are 'worst off' the initiatives hope to reduce the local health divide.

Providing intensive and sensitive tailored support

Another feature common to all of the projects is that they provide more intensive tailored support to individuals to achieve their goals. For example, in Stepping Out the project manager and clients design individual programmes of activities that are regularly reviewed and adapted. In the income maximisation project, individuals are identified and supported to apply for any benefits to which they are entitled but not receiving. One of the key aims of the education and training workstream in Leicestershire is to improve the sensitivity of services to particular groups' needs. Let's Get Serious is based on mentors' providing individual tailored support to schoolboys, but the mentors themselves also receive individual support from the project workers. In each of these projects the intensity and the focused nature of the support are argued to be key features of the project and vital to its success, given the significant needs of the individuals concerned.

Outreach

Finally, a number of the initiatives use different forms of outreach services to attempt to engage individuals who are otherwise often excluded from mainstream services. For example, the Leicestershire workstream is going out to local schools with ethnically diverse populations to encourage pupils to consider employment in the NHS. The income maximisation initiative has a number of particular strands, some of which directly contact disadvantaged people on GPs' lists, or go out to community centres to encourage people to think about their benefit entitlement.

Conclusion

The projects, described in much richer detail in the subsequent chapters, have much to commend them. As far as we can tell at this stage, each of the projects is making a real difference to the lives of people in disadvantaged circumstances, which will in time improve their health and could consequently reduce health inequalities. In terms of disseminating learning from their experiences, the detailed descriptions provided here do much to provide other places with ideas about different innovations to try in different contexts, and point out some of the problems that might be encountered and ways of avoiding them. Such information is extremely valuable. Moreover, the potential for learning from these projects will expand when their evaluations have been completed, so that we know if they have managed to achieve their goals and what aspects of these complex interventions have worked or not.

More broadly, the projects have a number of common characteristics, which have been suggested in reviews of successful interventions as being key to initiatives to address health inequalities (Schorr, 1988; Arblaster et al., 1996; Gunning-Schepers and Gepkens, 1996). Building on their individual successes, more focused evaluation and learning, which explore the contribution of these characteristics to achieving the projects' goals, will help to ensure that the innovative nature of their work is more clearly understood. In these ways more generalisable lessons would be possible and the pioneering efforts of these projects to explore new ways of improving the health of disadvantaged groups will contribute to the development of future initiatives and mainstream working to tackle health inequalities.

References

Acheson, D. (1998) *Independent inquiry into inequalities in health*, London: The Stationery Office.

Arblaster, L., Lambert, M., Entwistle, V., Forster, M., Fullerton, D., Sheldon, T. and Watt, I. (1996) 'A systematic review of the effectiveness of health service interventions aimed at reducing inequalities in health', *Journal of Health Services Research and Policy*, 1/2, 93–103.

Bauld, L., Judge, K., Lawson, L., Mackenzie, M., Mackinnon, J. and Truman, J. (2001) *Health Action Zones in transition: progress in 2000*, Glasgow: University of Glasgow.

Benzeval, M. and Meth, F. (2001) *Health inequalities: a priority at a crossroads*, draft report submitted to the Department of Health, November, London: Queen Mary, University of London.

Benzeval, M. and Meth, F. (2002), *Tackling inequalities in health: the HAZ way*, report submitted to the Department of Health, London: Queen Mary, University of London.

Denham, J. (1999) *Health Action Zones in 78 million pound trailblazing of 'money for modernisation': Zones will lead the way in modernising services and tackling inequalities*, press release 1999/0034, London: Department of Health.

Dobson, F. (1998) *Fifteen new Health Action Zones to tackle health inequalities*, press release 98/329, London: Department of Health.

DoH (2001) *Tackling health inequalities: consultation on a plan for delivery*, London: Department of Health.

Gunning-Schepers, L. and Gepkens, A. (1996) 'Reviews of interventions to reduce social inequalities in health: research and policy implications', *Health Education Journal*, 55, 226–38.

HAZ National Evaluation Team (1999) *Health Action Zones: learning to make a difference. Findings from a preliminary review of Health Action Zones and proposals for a national evaluation: a report submitted to the Department of Health*, PSSRU Discussion Paper 1546, June, Canterbury: University of Kent at Canterbury [available at http://www.ukc.ac.uk/PSSRU/downloads/ddp1546.html].

Jowell, T. (1999) *Health Action Zones are in the frontline in the war on health inequalities: trailblazers to report to ministers on action to drive up local standards of health*, press release 1999/0038, London: Department of Health.

Pawson, R. and Tilley, N. (1997) *Realistic evaluation*, London: Sage.

Schorr, L. (1988) *Within our reach: breaking the cycle of deprivation*, New York: Anchor.

CHAPTER 16

Modernisation and Health Action Zones: the search for coherence

Paul Crawshaw, Robin Bunton and Kate Gillen

Introduction

Modernisation has emerged as a key theme of HAZ policy, reflecting its growing importance within broader public policy debates. Recent government documents relating to the NHS (DoH, 1997, 2000) and social services (DoH, 1998) have stressed the need for modernisation across the public sector. As Powell (1999) notes, however, modernisation is an often used but rarely defined term in the vocabulary of the New Labour government (p. 336). Within the health service considerable emphasis has been placed upon the importance of 'modernising agendas' following the publication of *The NHS Plan* in July 2000 (DoH, 2000), and in earlier documents such as *The new NHS: modern, dependable* (DoH, 1997). This is evidenced by the creation of 'modernisation boards' to oversee the implementation of the NHS Plan within localities and the continual pressure to 'modernise services' from central government. Within the Teesside HAZ, which provides the empirical focus of this discussion, the theory and practice of modernisation have proved to be a contentious issue. Drawing upon an ongoing qualitative evaluation study, we examine the modernisation agenda in key stakeholders' reflections on HAZ process both locally and nationally.

Though present in the HAZ strategy from its outset, modernisation emerged with renewed vigour in 1999, and for many of those involved in the planning and implementation of the zones created something of a dilemma. As has been noted elsewhere in this collection, HAZs were initially conceived to address health inequalities in areas experiencing high levels of deprivation through implementing innovative projects, working in partnership and engaging communities. In early manifestations HAZs were understood as contributors to a broader agenda of NHS modernisation. As described in central government documentation, partnerships, collaboration and innovation are all understood as core to 'modern' government (Cabinet Office, 1999). If modernisation refers to 'joined-up working', creating alliances for innovative work to tackle deprivation and inequalities, from inception HAZs were 'modernisers'. However, the imposition of what has been described as a 'mainstream health service modernisation agenda' in 1999 has been felt to impact upon the HAZ through closer top-down monitoring of performance.

Modernisation in this new context is understood to refer to concentration upon NHS priority areas of community health development (CHD), cancer, mental health and waiting lists. The modernisation agenda focuses on more conventional health service targets and outcomes, and often seems incompatible with the original long-term strategies of partnership building and community empowerment, which are not necessarily measured by performance indicators. Investment in innovative working practices and 'bottom-up' community lead approaches are time-consuming and often difficult to assess by outcome measures. However, the impact of such work on hard to reach or particularly vulnerable groups can be significant. HAZs were understood to be an opportunity to develop such work and were felt by many to represent a shift towards a more 'public health' or 'whole systems' model of health care, seen as capable of addressing the broad determinants of health and tackling health inequalities. Some stakeholders involved in the Teesside HAZ suggest that the change in direction has led to fragmentation. Others suggest that a focus on mainstream health service agendas is a 'realistic' way of achieving targets for health improvement. This chapter uses empirical evidence collected with stakeholders involved in the Teesside HAZ to explore the impact of modernisation on one zone. Implications for the future of the national HAZ programme, and for health and social care policies and practices, are discussed.

The rise of modernisation

Notions of modernisation are not entirely new in public policy discourses and were a feature of previous Conservative government administrations (Grover and Stewart, 2000). Its re-emergence in recent Labour administration policy statements stresses its importance in developing strategies for improving public services across health, welfare and social care provision (see DoH, 1997, 1998, 2000). The precise meaning of the concept is far from clear, however. The use of the term 'modernisation' in policy discourses is at best complex and at worst highly ambiguous. A brief glance at the recent NHS Plan (DoH, 2000) shows the lack of clarity despite the frequency of use. From the outset the plan sets out to specify the aim of 'modernising the health service'. Here this is used in the literal sense of bringing it 'up to date', to be 'a 21st century health service'. It also uses modernisation in different ways to refer to patient- or user-centred services, enabling staff input into service development, and the achievement of new and more ambitious targets and outputs. Modernisation appears as a vehicle that will produce a renewed and reformed health service that, though committed to the traditional principles of equity and universalism, is prepared to change and develop in order to perform most efficiently and provide the best service for users. Blackman and Palmer (1999) suggest that modernisation refers to both centralisation and continuity with previous Conservative policies, thus reflecting Labour's 'third way' politics of pragmatism. This theme is reflected across the welfare sector as local authorities and providers strive to modernise and develop in order to come in line with new government agendas, focusing on perform-ance, accountability and efficiency, and new processes of scrutiny and target setting.

Modernisation, then, has many different meanings and is used in different ways in different contexts. Like other terms in social and public policy discourses it has become an essentially contested concept (Gallie, 1955–6; Plant et al., 1980) whose significance is clear, but meaning ambiguous. Its contested nature presents challenges for empirical study, but provides opportunity for critical reflection on how such initiatives are influenced by changing policy discourses, and how they are interpreted and implemented at a local level. Modernisation has been described in the NHS Plan (DoH, 2000) and local interpretations as 'redesigning the NHS around its patients and improving the lives of its staff – putting people at the centre of the system' (NHS Trent, 2001). Modernisation is also more generally described as a means of improving services by working towards national targets for health improvement such as: reducing waiting lists and the incidences of cancers, CHD, and focusing upon mental health. This focus upon centrally determined agendas and priorities has become the most significant manifestation of 'modernisation' in the Teesside HAZ. Many stake-holders involved in this zone feel that the removal of the bottom-up focus of the initiative restricted its original aim of providing local solutions to local problems. This finding is reflected in the national evaluation of the HAZ (see Bauld et al., 2001). Stakeholders suggest that the modernisation agenda has brought a focus on national targets and priorities at the expense of local autonomy and response to need. This is understood as a significant shift away from the original concep-tion of HAZs as representing decentralisation and local determination.

Methods

We report here on some of the findings of an evaluation process designed to explore HAZ implementation, development and delivery. This chapter draws on data from a series of qualitative interviews ($n = 102$) conducted with stakehold-ers involved in the Tees HAZ at both a planning and implementation level. These interviews took place over a 15 month period between April 2000 and June 2001, and generated a large amount of qualitative data. The material presented here represents only a small part of the overall study. Extracts presented are, however, representative of the views of the wider sample. At the time of writing (late 2001) the evaluation is ongoing and scheduled for completion by March 2002.

Modernisation and the Teesside HAZ

Originally Teesside HAZ was understood to be an initiative designed to tackle inequalities in health, with an emphasis upon partnerships and engaging communities. This was to be achieved by participation in innovative work, involving diverse providers in a 'public health' approach to health care which addressed the broad determinants of health. The emergence of the modernisation agenda has changed this direction. Emphasis upon performance has, for many stakeholders, stifled the potential for innovation and bottom-up community leadership.

Many respondents involved in the evaluation reported the fragmentation resulting from the redirection towards modernisation: 'The HAZ at this precise moment in time predominantly covers the modernisation agenda for the government which is a shift in direction from its initial concept. I now perceive it is purely there to drive the government's modernisation agenda.' The impact of the modernisation agenda on the zone is reiterated. There is, however, some ambiguity about the meaning of the term.

Some respondents discussed the modernisation of services in a similar manner to national policy documents, and suggested that these had guided the HAZ planning process: 'We looked at where current plans, whether it was national service framework or joint investment plans, had identified gaps where funding wasn't identified, where it could really make a difference, where it could meet the modernisation elements of the programme.' Other respondents suggested a shift away from the original conception of the HAZ as innovative and pioneering in using community development models:

> The modernisation agenda may cause some friction with the partners because they see that the government is encouraging a more mainstream approach. I think this is seen as a way of channelling the money into a more traditional way of commissioning health care and I think it could cause friction. The old regime is going to start pulling strings again.

This was felt to have impacted upon HAZ work in Teesside in a variety of ways:

> Last year they focused very much on improving health and health inequality. Now the modernisation agenda's come much more to the forefront. So now we're working towards both those remits really. So I think there's been a bit of confusion about the whole focus of the HAZ and what it is.

These sentiments are reflected in respondents' understandings of what the fundamental aims of the HAZ are or should be. Many felt these should be to work towards large-scale modernising projects, others to focus on the original emphasis of smaller-scale, more innovative pieces of work: 'We are told "We want large projects and we want them to work towards the modernising agenda". It means nothing to me really. If a small project works well why do I have to come up with large projects about modernising?'

Stakeholders consistently suggested that this problem of shifting agendas or 'moving goalposts' had created tensions and ambiguity at a local and national level between those directing policy and those implementing work on the ground. Respondents increasingly felt that modernisation would be the yardstick against which their achievements would be measured, over and above original aims of engaging communities and innovation: 'Our measurements are going to go against the national criteria for the modernisation agenda. Partnerships are in there, but I don't think that they are what we are being measured against. It's more access to services you know; cancer, mental health, CHD.'

Some stakeholders felt that this change was positive and contributed toward the overall HAZ aims of health improvement and tackling inequalities through creating potential to develop work and attract more funding: 'The national agenda has focused more and more on the issue of modernisation. It's been seen that you can create more capacity by using the HAZ as a building block to attract other sources of funding.' Others were more cynical, and suggested that this change in direction had moved the HAZ away from its initial focus which had been welcomed as a challenge to conventional models of service delivery: 'When [the HAZ] all came about everybody in health promotion was very excited. It was all about health promotion. Now it seems to have reverted to what it always is. Sort out sick people, the emphasis on waiting lists and clinical practice.'

The introduction of an agenda which had 'modernisation' as its key aim was thus understood to have caused fragmentation within the development and implementation of the HAZ in Teesside. Prioritising of national modernising agendas with a focus on more clinical outputs and conventional health service targets was felt to have stifled innovation in health promotion and disease prevention, and the potential for engaging communities in bottom-up solutions to health improvement.

Modernisation and national priorities

HAZs are accountable to regional NHS authorities which have subjected them to rigorous performance management processes. This has meant a high volume of administrative work and monitoring for those involved in both coordinating and implementing HAZ work. The shift towards the national priorities dictated by a modernisation agenda which required HAZs to focus on specific targets in their reporting and outputs for projects seems to have exacerbated this: 'Effectively what they're changing towards is you know addressing the HiMP [Health Improvement Programme] and Child Improvement Plan and reducing CHD, mental health and reducing fatal illness. They are the main focus because they are the main targets for the government.'

The shift in thinking locates HAZ more centrally within a modernisation agenda, and was felt to represent a significant move away from the original HAZ aims of innovation and change: 'Obviously it's changed a lot since I came into post. It's gone down a modernisation route and to be honest I think it will disappear'; 'I feel the excitement of health promotion being recognised and the importance of preventing ill health suddenly being overshadowed again.' This respondent refers to problems in project planning and implementation caused by the policy shift. Projects that had initially been conceived to address targets relating to local need and positing local solutions were increasingly compelled to address national priorities or risk losing their funding:

> The criteria changed to modernisation of services and when that happened there was a lot of frustration. If you had applied for three years' funding you were OK. But if you had only applied for one year's funding then you might have a project that was running quite well in the first year but because the criteria had changed they couldn't apply for further funding.

There was some concern among the HAZ community that these changes in policy had come about as part of a very much top-down process: 'In effect there was no control over the changing direction. It was a very top-down approach and I felt very strongly about that.'

The HAZ was seen to have undemocratically shifted from being a locally based programme able to identify and work towards local needs, to a more centrally driven initiative. Such tensions between local autonomy and central policies have been present in the health service since its inception (Klein, 1995), and it is therefore perhaps unsurprising that they have emerged within the HAZ programme. HAZs were initially intended, however, to be a different kind of initiative, with freedoms and flexibilities which would allow them to tackle local needs. Imposition of the modernisation agenda was experienced as a retrogressive return to national priorities.

As area-based initiatives or zones, HAZs reflect the New Labour administration's use of area targeting as a means of tackling problems associated with deprivation, inequality and exclusion. A key tenet of such zones is decentralisation and local autonomy in how budgets are spent and priorities addressed. This is reflected in other new area-based programmes such as Sure Start, New Deal for Communities and Education Action Zones, which attempt to use partnerships and community engagement as a mean of holistically addressing the catalogue of social problems characteristic of 'excluded' communities. The move within the HAZ to addressing more centrally driven agendas reflects a shift in the conception of such schemes, as monies initially intended to be spent on locally determined needs are here used for meeting regional and national health-improvement targets.

Although such an approach can bring benefits in terms of service provision for communities, their needs and expectations are not always congruent with those of policy makers. Those with direct involvement in communities are in a position to have a greater understanding of local needs and how these can be met. This may mean working in more innovative ways than conventional health-service-driven approaches allow: 'The disadvantage is that what the community wants often [isn't] the government's objectives. You go out and consult the community and what they want isn't five pieces of fruit a day, it's community safety.'

In their initial form HAZs were better equipped to manage this kind of 'innovative' approach to health improvement through establishing partnerships between diverse service providers and working with communities. Findings from our evaluation suggest that the shift towards modernisation and more limited health service priorities has stifled innovation, and required projects to be more mainstream and governed by 'top-down' agendas.

Modernisation and progress

Not all participants in our evaluation have viewed the growing influence of modernisation within the Teesside HAZ as a negative development. For others it was felt that the setting of targets and priorities more in line with traditional health service agendas was an appropriate way of tackling inequalities and improving services. These respondents suggested that a return to centrally driven dictates represented a way for them to use HAZ monies to achieve realistic targets with 'quantifiable' outputs, in contrast to pursuing what were represented as the less tangible goals of partnerships working and community engagement. As one respondent noted:

> I actually think it's more realistic. The NHS and social services are far too complex to be changed from a bottom-up approach with the size of the allocation we had. Little pockets of projects are not going to change this monster across Teesside. I think we have lost a bit of the bottom-up approach, but we will achieve more realistically.

The use of HAZ monies as a more 'mainstream' resource was understood by some stakeholders as a way of supplementing more conventional health service work already under way; thus the HAZ was seen as adding value to mainstream NHS provision and plugging gaps in existing services.

> We live in the real world, and there are targets that are quite rightly set about trying to tackle inequalities. The gaps in resources for mainstream health care in Teesside have been there for all to see. So it's quite right to be able to use significant sources of funding through the HAZ to repair those.

In this way a focus upon mainstream modernisation of services was understood as a more realistic way of tackling health inequalities and achieving health improvement for populations experiencing high levels of deprivation, with the resulting pressures upon local health services:

> I must admit I feel very strongly about the way it was set up at the beginning around small projects. The only advantage was that it produced quite a lot of innovative practice. The problem was that it was around little projects that didn't necessarily make a connection. So this focus around modernising the big money is more useful and is going to make a real difference.

It was suggested that the initial inception of HAZs, focused upon partnerships, engaging communities and innovation, was an unrealistic way of attempting to tackle health inequalities and that more mainstream health service agendas were an appropriate way to use HAZ monies to achieve targets: 'Some of the first-wave HAZ projects stretched the boundaries of health a bit more than I was comfortable with. As it has become more mainstream I have been able to use it more to develop things like mental health primary care.' Others suggested that it was more appropriate to work with a mixed economy model, using both innovative and conventional approaches:

> I think there is a tension around the previous model of empowering communities. The Department of Health has now been much more focused on the HAZ being used for bigger, more mainstream issues. That's created a tension but I think we are happy to live with that kind of mixed economy.

This 'mixed economy' has existed in Teesside as first-wave projects have endeavoured to maintain their emphasis on innovation and engaging communities. However, as noted in previous sections, this focus has to some extent been overshadowed by more mainstream agendas.

Discussion

Evidence from our ongoing evaluation suggests that the reintroduction of the modernisation agenda has had a significant impact on the Teesside HAZ, in a similar manner to elsewhere in the UK (Bauld et al., 2001). As a result, the work of the HAZ is being brought into line with the priorities for the 'new NHS' set out in various recent government documents.

Modernisation has become a key theme of recent UK government policy, and providers in health and social care and beyond have increasingly found themselves under pressure to contribute to a 'modernising' agenda. Modernisation is understood as relating to performance and efficiency, yet also to increased accessibility and transparency for users. For the NHS this means retaining a traditional focus upon equity and universalism while, simultaneously, working towards performance, efficiency and patient involvement. Such a conception of the 'modern' health service represents a continuation of some of the 'consumerist' rhetoric of previous Conservative administrations, while still maintaining traditional values, perhaps reflecting a 'third way', New Labour's pragmatism that eschews ideological commitment to beliefs of left and right policy agendas.

This model of service delivery has had a profound impact upon the HAZ. The need to meet targets which address conventional health service agendas has changed the 'bottom-up' focus of the zone, and this has been reflected in other zones around the UK (see Bauld et al., 2001). For the Teesside zone this has meant that some of the local energy for project work has been lost, and the potential to tackle problems in partnership with local communities has been reduced. This is significant as HAZs, and other area-based programmes such as the New Deal for Communities and Sure Start, are designed to meet local needs, to be responsive to community voices and allow innovation, even straying beyond conventional service provision. What is understood by modernisation appears to work in the opposite direction and is often experienced as disruptive and confusing. If future area-based programmes are to be successful 'trailblazers' working with communities to improve services and reduce inequalities, they will need the freedoms and flexibilities to fend off the shifting, top-down, central policy developments such as 'the modernisation agenda', as pressures to meet centrally defined performance targets have, for many of our respondents, stifled innovation and the potential to work towards sustainable, bottom-up, community-determined health solutions.

References

Bauld, L., Judge, K., Lawson, L., Mackenzie, M., Mackinnon, J. and Truman, J. (2001) *Health Action Zones in transition: progress in 2000*, Glasgow: University of Glasgow.

Blackman, T. and Palmer, A. (1999) 'Continuity or modernisation? The emergence of New Labour's welfare state', in Dean, H. and Woods, R. (eds), *Social Policy Review 11*, Luton: Social Policy Association, 107–26.

Cabinet Office (1999) *Modernising government*, London: The Stationery Office.

DoH (1997) *The new NHS: modern, dependable*, London: The Stationery Office.

DoH (1998) *Modernising social services*, London: The Stationery Office.

DoH (2000) *The NHS Plan*, London: The Stationery Office.

Gallie, W. B. (1955–6) 'Essentially contested concepts', *Proceedings of the Aristotelian Society*, 56, 157–97.

Grover, C. and Stewart, J. (2000) 'Modernising social security? Labour and its welfare-to-work strategy', *Social Policy and Administration*, 34/3, 235–52.

Klein, R. (1995) *The new politics of the NHS*, London: Longman.

NHS Trent (2001) *What is modernisation?*, Sheffield: NHS Executive Trent [available at http://www.nhsetrent.gov.uk/modernisation/whatis.htm].

Plant, K., Lesser, H. and Gooby, P. (1980) *Political philosophy and social welfare: essays on the normative basis of welfare provision*, London: Routledge.

Powell, M. (1999) 'New Labour and the third way in the British National Health Service', *International Journal of Health Services*, 29/2, 353–70.

CHAPTER 17

The pain and exhilaration of innovation

Richard Strittmatter and Michael Stores

Let's Get Serious Ltd is a Health Action Zone Innovations Fund Project, managed by the National HAZ Innovations Fund Manager, operating within the Manchester, Salford and Trafford Health Action Zone. The project aims to train and employ up to 30 unemployed men to provide a network of support for boys and young men that are at risk of being marginalised because of antisocial behaviour, educational underachievement or drug use. The aim is to improve health, both mental and physical; reduce self-harm from drugs and alcohol among both groups; provide emotional and educational support for the boys; and, at the same time, give the men both training and employment opportunities.

The project also attempts to tackle the root causes of the health inequalities facing unemployed men. The problems that unemployed men experience often have a profound impact on their self-esteem and self-confidence at one end of the scale, through to serious depression and high young male suicide rates. LGS's pioneering holistic approach seeks to address all of these issues.

This chapter describes the origins of the Let's Get Serious project and outlines the progress made in its first year. The chapter begins with an outline of the context of the project – the core priorities which it aims to address. It then describes how the project was implemented, and concludes with a summary of some of the progress made thus far.

Core priorities

Let's Get Serious aims to provide unemployed men with an opportunity to act as mentors for young men and boys at risk of exclusion and disadvantage. In doing this it is focusing on the reduction of four prevalent problems: poor mental health and suicide; poor health; poor educational attainment; and crime.

Mental health and suicide

The Department of Health report entitled *Children and adolescents who try to harm, hurt or kill themselves* (DoH, 2001) has thrown up some disturbing findings. Approximately 2.1% of 11–15-year-olds have tried to harm, hurt or even kill themselves. The rate of self-harm among the 11–15-year-olds with no mental disorder was 1.2%. This rate increases noticeably to 9.4% for those affected by anxiety disorders.

Suicide is the biggest killer among men aged between 15 and 35, accounting for 21% of all deaths among this age group in Britain. Suicide rates among young men have been increasing over the last 20 years: between 1971 and 1997 the suicide death rate for men aged 15 to 24 rose from 6.9 per 100,000 to 16.4 per 100,000 population. In 1999, of 24 deaths in Manchester in the age group 15–24, a quarter were determined as suicide or undetermined injury, according to Office for National Statistics (ONS) mortality figures (ONS, 1999). Suicide rates among men in Manchester and Salford are the worst in the country, over 60% higher than the national average for the age range 15–34 (ibid.).

According to the Policy Studies report *Youth unemployment, labour market programmes and health* (Lakey et al., 2001), being out of work can make existing problems seem worse. Jobless people are more likely to have lower levels of general health, with higher levels of anxiety and depression. Unemployment is a significant risk factor in suicides: one in seven men will develop a depressive illness within the first six months of unemployment, while long-term unemployment is associated with a doubling of the male suicide rate.

It has been suggested that the biggest obstacle to tackling male mental health issues, including suicide, is men themselves, and in particular their reluctance to talk about their feelings. In a national opinion poll carried out for the Samaritans, 84% of men polled said that they felt ashamed or embarrassed when simply talking about their emotions (Katz et al., 1999). Depression and mental health issues carry enormous stigma, particularly when it's men who are suffering from them. Very little has been published about the relationship between masculinity and suicide, although tentative links are sometimes alluded to. There has been some speculation that adolescent and young men are particularly vulnerable to mental health problems because of feelings of inadequacy, or 'not measuring up as a man', during this stressful period of their lives.

Other factors can also be significant. Substance misuse has long been recognised as a risk factor for suicide: alcohol and other drugs can affect reasoning, and they can lower inhibitions and so make suicide attempts more likely.

Health

The average person in Manchester lives several years less than their peers in other parts of the UK. Life expectancy charts published by the Office for National Statistics (DoH, 1999) reveal wide variations from region to region between the years 1997 and 1999. In Manchester, men live to approximately 70 years, compared to the national average of about 75 years. Men who live in the Manchester Health Authority area die the earliest, at just over 70 years; by contrast, men who reside in the Kensington, Chelsea and Westminster Health Authority can expect to live for over 78.64 years. By comparison, the national average life expectancy for women is just over 80 years: the figure for Manchester is 76.22 years, and the best in England and Wales is 83.08 years, in Kensington, Chelsea and Westminster.

Men are more likely to smoke, to have a poor diet and to be overweight than women. In addition, they are three times more likely than women to be alcohol dependent, and four times as likely to be registered drug addicts. Even so, men are about half as likely to visit their doctor compared to women. Coronary heart disease (CHD) is one of the main causes of death in the UK, and death rates from CHD are among the highest in the world, according to British Heart Foundation figures (British Heart Foundation, 2000). CHD kills one in four men and one in five women in Great Britain.

In the UK more cancer deaths can be attributed to smoking than to any other risk factor. The proportion of smokers is higher in the manual socioeconomic groups than among those in non-manual groups. Statistics published in the ONS general household survey (ONS, 1998) show that the percentage of men and women smoking in the North-West region is higher than the national average for England. Despite the downward general trend in cigarette smoking, the rate in the North-West remains slightly higher than the national average. The teen smoking attitudes survey (DoH, 2000) carried out in 1998 on a group of 11–15-year-olds showed that 10% were regular smokers. Smoking activity increases with age: while less than 1% of 11-year-olds were regular smokers, over 21% of 15-year-olds were.

Education

Pupils in the Manchester and Salford Local Education Authority areas perform significantly below the national average. In addition, girls routinely outperform boys. Some key statistics are presented in Tables 17.1 and 17.2. As the tables illustrate, educational attainment in terms of key stage 3 assessment test results and GCSE passes is considerably lower in the Manchester Salford and Trafford area than nationally.

Table 17.1 Key stage 3 assessment test results: percentage of pupils achieving level 5 or above

	English (%)		Mathematics (%)		Science (%)	
	Boys	Girls	Boys	Girls	Boys	Girls
England	56	73	65	67	66	65
Manchester	43	60	46	52	46	48
Salford	48	67	54	62	55	59
Trafford	68	80	72	74	73	72

Source: figures derived from the DfES (2001b).

Crime

There is a popular misconception about the amount of offences that are attributable to young people. For example, 76% of detected crime in 1999 was committed by people over the age of 18, and people over 21 were responsible for almost 60% of detected offences (Nacro, 1999).

Table 17.2 Percentage of pupils achieving five or more GCSE passes (grades A–C)

	5+ GCSEs (%)
England	50.0
Manchester	31.0
Salford	34.3
Trafford	57.7

Source: Figures derived from DfES (2001a).

Young frequent and heavy drinkers are more likely to become victims of some form of crime, often violent, as well as to commit minor violent crime themselves. The relationship between alcohol consumption and offending has been analysed using approximately six hundred 17–21-year-old males sentenced to detention in a young offender institution. Significantly, the figures show that 41% of the sample reported being drunk or having drunk alcohol at the time of their current offence (Cookson, 1992).

There is also increasing evidence showing that young offenders are at high risk of both involvement with drugs and of developing problematic drug use. It suggests that drug misusers are more likely to be involved with other forms of offending. The Audit Commission report *Misspent youth* (Audit Commission, 1999) showed that 15% of young offenders had a drug problem of some kind, and this number increased to 37% among the more persistent offenders.

According to a study of drug use and smoking among teenagers published by the ONS (DoH, 2000), alcohol is the most common drug used by young people. The numbers of 14–15-year-olds using drugs has increased six-fold since 1987. Figures also indicate that people are trying drugs at a younger age. By comparison, the percentage of 12–13-year-olds who had tried drugs in 1996 is actually higher than the percentage of 15–16-year-olds who had tried drugs in 1987 (Balding, 1999). Regular consumption of alcohol often starts at an early age: 89% of children admit to having had their first alcoholic drink by the age of 13 (Royal College of Physicians, 1995). Alcohol abuse among young people can lead to a variety of problems, such as poor school achievement, unsociable behaviour, truancy, unemployment, problems with relationships and delinquency.

Implementing the initiative

The first group of Let's Get Serious trainee mentors (12 in total) were recruited in December 2000; all were previously unemployed. Each trainee studied for an accredited mentoring course, equivalent to an NVQ level 3.

The trainees work in their placements for three days per week, and come in to the LGS offices on the other two days. The trainees have regular supervision interviews with their line manager, as well as participating in full team meetings to give them an opportunity to discuss their work with their peers. The trainee mentors will continue to receive ongoing training and support throughout their time with LGS. In addition, the trainee mentors will be taught a variety of skills, including presentation skills, so they can act as advocates for the project, as well as increase their own confidence. The trainees will study for a certificate in counselling, and learn IT and other relevant skills.

The mentors offer troubled young people time and space in a nonjudgemental way to look at some of their difficulties, and to encourage and support their involvement in a variety of activities, such as photography, music or sport. The aim is to increase the young people's self-esteem, which in turn may lead to educational and other life-style improvements.

Selecting trainees

The selection criteria used to recruit the first group of trainees have been the subject of much discussion, and in fact a number of changes were made to the criteria used to recruit the second group of mentors. These criteria may be reviewed after the intake of the next group of trainees to ensure that the best candidates are selected, though the LGS board of directors has expressed concerns regarding the exclusion of too many candidates if the selection criteria are not exactly right.

In accordance with Home Office circular 47/1993, *Access to children checks*, the trainee mentors were subjected to stringent police checks. The safeguards have two elements, one of which is the police check; the other is a local authority inspection. Clearly, checks are essential particularly when the trainee mentors will be working with young people, but the consequent hold-ups can be extremely frustrating and difficult to accept, particularly when one authority moves much quicker than another. LGS has now had some initial meetings with the authorities which grant approval to see if the process can be speeded up, and to establish exactly where any problems may lie.

The decision to appoint mentors with a wide variation in age, background, educational ability and culture was laudable as an attempt to represent the diversities of the cultures in which the organisation is operating. The trainees all have experience of the pressures of living in inner city areas, and gained the confidence of their peers and mentees by having shared background, shared experiences and common values.

Training

The diversity of the group led to a number of issues emerging. It had been hoped that the mentors would complete their training within a six-month period. It is now evident that the timescale requires revision, as it took some of the trainee mentors almost twice as long as envisaged to complete the course. A knock-on effect was that the appointment of the next cohort had to be postponed until the first group were trained and working in satisfactory placements. A review of the recruitment and selection procedure is currently taking place, discussions are ongoing at board level regarding refining the criteria by which candidates are selected, and it may be that a test will be included during the selection procedure to ensure that candidates have the ability to study to the required level.

HAZ executive director Edna Robinson is sanguine:

> If it takes longer than we thought for some of these newly employed men to gain their confidence and their competence, that is fine. This agency is a public service and we are here to develop their self-esteem – which is an outcome in itself. Their employability is a second outcome and their effectiveness is a third outcome, so we've got a win–win–win situation.

Work placements

A further issue that arose from the diverse nature of the first intake of trainee mentors concerned the practice of securing work placements. With the completion of their training, the mentors were found work placements in a variety of organisations, schools, sports clubs and youth offending teams, for example. A number of organisations sympathetic to the aims of Let's Get Serious very kindly offered to take on the trainees. Some of the organisations went out on a limb to take on the trainees, and have been supportive of the mentors and the project, which would have run into real difficulties without the support of these organisations.

In general it was easier to obtain placements for the older mentors than the younger mentors. The reasons for the popularity of the elder mentors can be guessed at – more life experience to draw on, greater maturity and so on. A deliberate decision was made to employ a diverse group of young men, and so if the younger members are more difficult to place, then recruitment and selection guidelines may have to be revised, or extra training may need to be given to the younger trainees. The board has discussed this situation, and a lower age limit may be introduced for the second group of trainees. However, to alleviate worries about exclusion, the age limit will be subject to a degree of flexibility, and will be reviewed following the recruitment of the second group of trainees.

Some of the trainees working in schools have expressed some dissatisfaction with the way in which they have been used. They have expressed the opinion that they are being used as classroom assistants rather than using their mentoring skills to help pupils and students. Teachers, of course, are under pressure to deliver the curriculum and to meet their targets, so it is no surprise that teaching staff want to use the trainees to support curriculum delivery. As to the purpose of the mentors, the trainees want to develop their counselling skills but not necessarily in a classroom environment. It has become apparent that a tighter set of guidelines may be needed to inform schools of the skills and expectations of the mentors, and that Let's Get Serious may need to liaise more closely with schools and teachers.

Mentees

Mentees come to LGS from a variety of routes. Some of the trainee mentors are working in schools, and so typically mentees are referred to them by the teaching staff. However, there is an element of self-referral, because the young people know that LGS mentors are in the building at certain times in the week, and can choose to go and see them at those times. This can occasionally lead to workload problems.

Let's Get Serious mentors have also been working with young people referred by local youth offending teams. In common with the experience elsewhere, there is also a degree of self-referral whereby young people choose to go to see the mentors whenever they are available. LGS has also mentees referred by other agencies, such as the Millennium Awards, Family Support Units, Lifeline and other voluntary organisations, as well as receiving enquiries from individuals. In fact, at times there is more demand than LGS currently satisfies.

Supporting trainees

There have been pressures regarding LGS's role employing and supporting a vulnerable and disaffected client group, and the aspirations of the project in terms of wanting to convey a thoroughly professional and dynamic image. Some of the trainees have required additional support to achieve the standard for accreditation, and need more personal support than some of the other more successful trainees. LGS aims to help individuals from all kinds of backgrounds, and with a wide range of experience and abilities. It also wants to be seen as a vibrant organisation offering a professional service, and at times there are conflicting pressures that need resolving. The two aspirations are not incompatible, but the tensions that exist between them need sensitive management to ensure that equilibrium is maintained.

Only one of the trainees has decided to leave the project completely, which is an outstanding retention rate given the challenging background of some of the trainee mentors. In fact, the individual who decided to leave LGS is now in employment, and although his departure was a loss to LGS his achievement in subsequently securing work is a real success. One factor that prompted his leaving was that he didn't enjoy working with young people. The board has discussed this situation, and in future the recruitment and selection procedure may be revised to try to ensure that candidates are willing to work with young people. Let's Get Serious is also considering offering a broader range of opportunities, because clearly not everyone is suited to a counselling or mentoring role.

The Let's Get Serious project has unfortunately received some negative press coverage. One local paper ran the headline 'Ex-cons to "mentor" kids', and focused on the salary that the trainee mentors are being paid. In fact, it costs approximately £1000 per week to keep one young person in local authority secure accommodation; prison on average costs £25,000 per year per prisoner; and the average cost of a community punishment is around £2000. Figures provided by Payback (2001) show that prison sentences are no more effective than community punishments at preventing re-offending –approximately 80% of convicted offenders will re-offend. Let's Get Serious received just under £2 million for three years' funding from the HAZ Innovations Fund: if the mentors work with approximately ten young people and the young people and the mentors are kept out of the justice system, then the money that LGS receives looks to be well spent.

Let's Get Serious should be looked at not just in financial terms, but also in terms of the social costs if nothing is done to address the problems faced by young people in the region. It is difficult for the trainee mentors to disengage from inappropriate activities and to resist negative pressures, and it is to the individual's and the project's great credit that they have managed to do so. The act of employing the trainees can also have positive effects: the local economy receives a boost, benefiting from the new-found spending power of the formerly long-term unemployed mentors.

There have been a number of minor work-related concerns, regarding timekeeping, sickness reporting, annual leave and so on. These concerns were anticipated and have been dealt with in-house; copies of the company's policies concerning working practices have been distributed to all trainees, who have been reminded of their responsibilities. It is worth remembering that many of these young men have experienced long periods of unemployment, and so it may take them some time to get used to the working culture, and the rules and regulations of working life.

Progress

The project is now approximately 12 months old and entering its 'difficult' second phase. LGS is preparing to take on a second group of trainees. There have inevitably been some teething problems, some of which are detailed above, but given the innovative nature of the project, difficulties were not unexpected.

Let's Get Serious has recently been visited by the HAZ National Evaluation Team, based at Birmingham University, which has provided the project with a reporting framework to work to in the future. The informal feedback so far has been very encouraging. LGS is also just about to commission some research regarding the project's impact on health, and its long-term financial viability. The mentors' personal development is well documented via their regular one-to-ones with their line manager.

The positive effects on the first group of trainee mentors are evident (see Box 17.1): they are more confident and outgoing, they have acquired new knowledge and skills, and they have new purpose and resiliency. The mentors strive to be professional in any situation: they are as unfazed by MPs and radio interviews as they are by 12-year-old mentees. They have a much more healthy life style than formerly and a much greater awareness of health issues, and they contribute to the local economy in which they work. In fact, they act as advocates for the project far more effectively than any officer or any report.

Box 17.1 Case studies (names have been changed)

LGS gave 21-year-old Daniel his first ever job interview. Previously, Dan had been involved in voluntary work with a local drugs charity, Lifeline. 'Somebody suggested I'd be good at this job because of my own experience of problems. That's made me feel a bit better about myself,' he explains, adding: 'My parents and friends are seeing a change in my attitude altogether. I feel like a different person. I feel better, more confident.'

'My problems started in primary school,' says Adam, a trainee mentor with Let's Get Serious. 'I got expelled at the age of seven, though I was bright and had a lot of potential. It was due to lack of attention. I think guys crave attention, especially young boys. We were in the same situation as the kids we are going to help now. We've been there, in that scene. Maybe if I'd had a mentor when I was a young man I would have progressed better.'

LGS has begun to tackle the social exclusion faced by the mentors. The mentors are now endeavouring to contribute to tackling inequalities among the communities in which they work. If the LGS model is judged a success then it could perhaps be 'franchised out' and applied country-wide. In addition, Let's Get Serious is actively seeking funding to establish a female version of the project. The aims of LGS link the work of the Department of Health, Home Office, Department for Education and Skills, and the Department for Work and Pensions. As such, it provides a positive example of a joined-up community-based project in action.

References

Audit Commission (1999) *Misspent youth '99: the challenge for youth justice*, London: Audit Commission.

Balding, J. (1999) *Young people and illegal drugs in 1998*, Exeter: Schools Health Education Unit.

British Heart Foundation (2000) *It'll never happen to me*, British Heart Foundation.

Cookson, H. (1992) 'Alcohol use and offence type in young offenders', *British Journal of Criminology*, 32/3, 352–60.

DfES (2001a) *GCSE/GNVQ and GCE A/AS/Advanced GNVQ results for young people in England, 2000–2001 (provisional)*, November, Office for National Statistics.

DfES (2001b) *National Curriculum assessments of 7, 11 and 14 year olds by local education authority, 2001*, Statistical First Release, October, London: Department for Education and Skills.

DoH (1999) *Life expectancy at birth (years) and rank order by health authority in England and Wales*, Office for National Statistics.

DoH (2000) *Drugs use, smoking and drinking among young teenagers in 1999*, Office for National Statistics.

DoH (2001) *Children and adolescents who try to harm, hurt or kill themselves*, Office for National Statistics.

Katz, A., Buchanan, A. and McCoy, A. (1999) *Young men speak out*, London: Samaritans.

Lakey, J., Mukherjee, A. and White, M. (2001) *Youth unemployment, labour market programmes and health: a review of the literature*, London: Policy Studies Institute.

Nacro (2001) *Some facts about young people who offend*, Youth Crime Factsheet, London: Nacro [available at http://www.nacro.org.uk/].

ONS (1998) *Living in Britain: results from the general household survey*, Office for National Statistics.

ONS (1999) *VS3: mortality statistics (deaths by cause, age and sex)*, Office for National Statistics.

Payback (2001) *Rough guide to sentencing* [available at http://www.payback.org.uk/attitudes_to_punishment.html].

Royal College of Physicians (1995) *Alcohol and young people*, London: Royal College of Physicians and British Paediatric Association.

CHAPTER 18

An evaluation of benefits advice in primary care: Camden and Islington Health Action Zone

Salma Burton and David Diaz de Leon

Background

It has been well established through previous studies that there exists a link between social deprivation and health status. These variations in health status are influenced by a number of factors, such as home location, social class, career and ethnicity. People can be seen to be deprived if they lack the material standards of diet; clothing; housing; household facilities; working, environmental and locational conditions; and facilities which are ordinarily available to their society. They can be deprived if they do not participate in or have access to the forms of employment, occupation, education, recreation, and family and social activities and relationships which are commonly experienced or accepted (Acheson, 1998).

Among the most deprived groups in the Camden and Islington area of London are ethnic minorities and refugees, older pensioners and the disabled (Camden and Islington Health Authority, 2001). For members of the population with low income, who are more likely to suffer deprivation, the reliance on welfare benefits is crucial. However, it is widely known that many people, in particular the elderly, either do not claim or under-claim benefits due to them (Costigan et al., 1999). As a result people live on incomes that are lower than they are entitled, with their wellbeing subsequently negatively affected.

Since 1999 the Health Action Zone (HAZ) has funded six projects that were aimed at improving the health of the people living in Camden and Islington by increasing their income. These projects built their foundation on the theory that increasing income will improve people's health. The strategies used in the projects focused on increasing people's income by giving benefits advice and welfare rights advice. The projects were: Benefits Advice in Primary Care in South Islington; Benefits Advice in Primary Care in North Islington; Benefits Advice in Primary Care in South Camden; Income Maximisation for Older People in

Camden; Income Maximisation for Older People in Islington; and Income Maximisation in Kilburn. The objectives of these project were:

- to increase access to benefits advice
- to increase the income from benefits for people who are not currently receiving their full entitlement
- to improve people's health status by increasing their income.

The projects

Benefits Advice in Primary Care in South Islington

This project was started in December 1999 and involves provision of benefits advice in general practitioner (GP) surgeries. It was built on the experience of Islington People's Rights (IPR), which provides benefits advice and support, as well as managing the project with support from the South Islington Primary Care Group (PCG). The project was set up to enable all residents of the South Islington PCG area to have access to welfare rights advice in a doctor's surgery near their home. The service aims to utilise the cooperation of primary health care teams, the voluntary sector and social services. Many of the sessions are open to other residents whose GP practices do not host a welfare rights service.

Currently 10 sessions are held in 9 of the 16 practices that host the service. The HAZ funded the project for two years with just over £50,000 a year. During the period January to December 2000, 364 advice sessions were held in the various practices. Altogether 1761 appointments were booked, with a high attendance rate – higher than that for GP appointments. A total of 1388 clients were seen during the first year. On average just over 50% of clients were from ethnic minorities.

Benefits Advice in Primary Care in North Islington

Similar to the South Islington project, this project in North Islington also aimed at providing all needy residents of North Islington PCG area an opportunity to access benefits advice in a doctor's surgery near their home. This project was started in August 2000 and the service is currently hosted in five practices. During the first six months approximately 465 people were either seen or interviewed by telephone to assess their knowledge of welfare rights.

Benefits Advice in Primary Care in South Camden

The South Camden Benefits Advice for Primary Care project is based at Somers Town Medical Centre – a new GP practice on Chalton Street. The project started in January 2001, and was intended to focus on providing benefits advice to families with young children who have a significant health deficit. The aim of this project was to work with GPs and other primary care staff to identify priority groups and work with individuals to maximise their income from benefits available. The project was based on previous work of the Camden Citizens Advice Bureau (CAB) programme at the Caversham Group Practice's Primary Care for Older People Project.

The HAZ invested £25,000 in this project. The surgery wrote to 135 different patients on the practice list introducing them to the service. Of the 96 patients interviewed, 69 (72%) were taken onto the register of benefits advisers; 64% of these people are Bangladeshi.

Income Maximisation for Older People in Camden

This project, implemented by Camden Welfare Rights, used a strategic approach and had several components, including outreach work, joint work with the benefits division, benefits awareness training for staff and developing a benefits guide for older people. The focus of the project was to promote benefits take-up and income maximisation, and to identify the barriers to claiming benefits faced by older people. As part of this project, outreach work for the over-65 population was conducted in Ingestre Road Community Centre with their Good Neighbour Scheme, Hillwood Centre and the Millman Centre. The project also made links with other community organisations.

During the one year of HAZ funding (£18,869), 325 older people were offered benefits advice through the various initiatives undertaken. Following specialist help over 20% of them received extra benefits, with many claimants doubling their weekly income. The annual benefits gain has been recorded as £114,000, with a number of claims still outstanding. The project had also promoted joint working between the voluntary and statutory sectors, including work with the Welfare Rights Unit, CAB, Age Concern, Housing Benefits, Benefits Agency, local community centres and the Good Neighbour Scheme.

Income Maximisation for Older People in Islington

This project is located in the Whittington Hospital and includes outreach work. The project started in July 2000. Initial project activities included discussions with the hospital departments to identify the elderly Islington patients needing income support to refer them to the advice worker. The hospital department currently hosts the benefits service and does referrals. Initial activities also included preparing a briefing pack to 'sell' the project and briefing sessions for frontline staff. The service operates through social workers referring patients to the advice worker. The advice worker then visits patients, sometimes in hospital and often at home, to provide the advice and support needed in order to maximise the client's income.

The HAZ invested £15,000 in this project. Since the inception of the programme, an average of four referrals a day are made in the hospital, and over 30 clients have been seen by the advice worker at their homes. All the home visits resulted in benefits claims.

Income Maximisation in Kilburn

The purpose of this project was to provide outreach income-maximisation advice at various community locations in the Kilburn and Priory wards of Camden. Weekly income-maximisation sessions are held in community centres, and one-off sessions were previously held at various community centres in the Camden ward. From the 259 clients contacted in the second year a total of 475 inquiries were generated over the course of the project. The majority of inquiries were benefit-related, and 66 were related to debt. In total, 115 income increases were identified. The total output so far of the project includes 252 new client issue assessments, 115 income increases identified, 47 specialist advocacy referrals, and 6 promotions/campaigns. The project was designed to get as many people advice as possible; however, many of the clients were repeat callers with separate issues.

Purpose of evaluation and methodology

The need to evaluate these benefits advice/welfare rights related projects of the HAZ was identified by the HAZ Underlying Causes Programme Planning group. The core activities of the evaluation were conducted during June and July 2001.

The short duration of these projects dictated the methodology for evaluation. The methodology chosen acknowledged the difficulty of attributing changes in clients' health status to these projects, as well as the difficulty of attributing overall changes in health status of individuals who received welfare advice. There have been other similar projects implemented in Camden and Islington during the period. Since the projects were based on the evidence that increases in income reduces ill health, the extent to which incomes have increased was a focus of this evaluation. We also examined the processes by which income maximisation was achieved, and the extent to which the projects were effective.

The evaluation had to capture the value of rather short-term projects – some of them completed, others that were only just initiated. The projects also used different approaches. As a result, all the projects had to be examined within their contexts. We were careful not to directly compare the projects because of their inherent differences. While some (for instance, North and South Islington) used similar approaches, they operated in different circumstances, and it was determined inappropriate to analyse and compare the projects in isolation from the context and the circumstances in which they operated.

We attempted a high level of involvement of the stakeholders of the projects in the evaluation. We also ensured that evaluation was conducted in such a way that it would enable and enhance use of the evaluation findings. The objectives of the evaluation were agreed through initial discussions with project leads. They were:

- to identify the value of the income-maximisation services in the HAZ
- to assess the most appropriate ways in which income-maximisation services could be provided
- to identify lessons that could be learnt in order to inform future planning.

Methods used included the preliminary meetings with project leads, and the review of project monitoring, and other documents and related literature and interviews, with project leads, senior officials of the various organisations, representatives of implementing agencies, such as the Citizens Advice Bureau, front-line workers, including advice workers, and some clients. Questionnaires were sent to all the GP practices in Islington. The information collected was analysed to answer key questions agreed by the project leads:

- What are the obstacles to claiming benefits?
- How effective were the projects?
- What is the best approach to providing the service?
- What are the obstacles to providing the service?
- How important is this service?

Obstacles to claiming

This research identified several barriers to claiming benefits. Some of the barriers related to people's attitude to claiming, while others related to the process of claiming. Both types of barriers were also found to be interrelated, and the elderly and ethnic minority groups were found to be most affected by these barriers. Complex claim systems, frequent changes in the claim system and lengthy forms as long as 48 pages to be filled have been major obstacles to claiming benefits experienced by the elderly, ethnic minorities and the population in general.

The elderly in particular often also had a negative attitude towards claiming. Many of them saw claiming as 'scrounging' on the state, and felt they were taking money that could be helping more disadvantaged people. They felt guilty about accepting money they had not earned. Also, the sense of 'stigma' attached to claiming added to the reasons for not claiming, especially in conjunction with a complex claims process. The elderly found processes such as queuing, providing personal details on forms and the process of having to fill in forms not just difficult to undertake but also an 'intrusion on their privacy'. Previous refusal hindered people from attempting to claim again, even when it was clear to advice workers that claims were likely to be successful.

Effectiveness of the service

In examining how effective delivery of benefits advice service through the six HAZ projects have been, the following issues were examined.

Demand for the service

The findings of this study clearly revealed that there was a distinct and increasing demand for the service. As information on the existence of the service disseminated through word of mouth and official means, the client numbers increased significantly. For instance, in the case of the South Islington project, in the first six months 4.2 clients were booked. This number exceeded the 3 bookings per session expected. In the second six months the demand increased to 5.3 bookings per session.

The number of clients seen and the number of claims made depended on the nature of claims, the target population of the project, and the duration and scale of the project. In the case of the South Islington project a total of 1388 clients were seen in the first year. In the South Camden primary care project, where the service is being delivered in one GP practice, 96 people were interviewed during the first six months; 69 of these (64% from the Bangladeshi community) took up the service.

Increase in client incomes

One of the most significant findings of the study was the remarkable increase in client incomes. In the Camden Income Maximisation for Older People project, £9954 invested in the benefits advice services delivered by the Camden Citizens Advice Bureau generated client incomes of a total of £103,840.44. Camden

CAB estimates that the £25,000 a year invested by the HAZ will increase the annual total income of the clients of this project by over £270,000. On the whole it was possible to conclude that for every £10,000 invested in benefits advice service delivery, there was a £100,000 increase every year of clients' total incomes.

Success of the projects was demonstrated by information on the number of clients seen by the different services, the number of people who claimed, the number of successful claims and the amount of additional income generated. Having established this, it was then necessary to find out which of the project approaches were most effective in delivering benefits advice services.

Best approach to providing the service

Benefits advice services provided across the six HAZ-funded projects have been either GP practice based, GP practice based with home visits, hospital based with home visits, or outreach work via community centres – advice and home visits, and provision of information and training. The wide-ranging differences in the duration and value as well as the approaches used meant that it was difficult to identify the most effective or successful project. However, we found that that the Camden Income Maximisation for Older People project used the most strategic approach. The South Islington primary care project was the most effective in terms of providing a service to a wider target population, and demonstrated the outstanding capacity of Islington People's Rights to provide efficient and coordinated services. In comparison the North Islington primary care project not only started late but encountered many problems that could be clearly linked to the number of single-handed GP practices with limited staff, capacity and space for hosting benefits advice services.

In this evaluation we attempted to identify the best approach for providing a benefits advice service. The finding was that no single approach should be used. However, the GP practice based approach rated highest in terms of delivering the service to a wide range of people. Targeted services – such as home visits, community-based information (as in the case of the elderly) and borough-based information dissemination in different languages to keep communities, particularly ethnic minorities, informed of benefits system changes and welfare rights services – were found to be important in order to reach the most deprived people.

Obstacles to providing the service

At the initial meetings with project leads it was clear that some of the projects faced various obstacles during the initial stages of establishment. For instance, for various reasons some took time to be implemented. There were also concerns that GPs are against hosting a benefits advice service, possibly because it would increase their workload and attract the 'wrong patients'. This evaluation attempted to clarify the validity of these concerns.

Through questionnaires sent to all the GP practices in Islington, with a response rate of 68%, we established that none of these practices were concerned about attracting the 'wrong patients'. Only two of the practices stated they do not wish to host a benefits advice service, but attributed this to the shortage of staff, capacity and space. On the whole it was found that GP practices would host benefits advice services if they were supported with extra resources. In South Islington, which has a smaller number of larger (group) practices, project leads found it easier to host the services, whereas in North Islington, where many GP practices work single-handed, it was more difficult to establish the service. In the case of some service providers it was also found that lack of, or limited, capacity to provide an efficient service hindered the project's success.

Importance of the service

Evaluations of HAZ projects are conducted with the purpose of identifying evidence of success and disseminating the findings in order to inform the mainstreaming of HAZ projects, particularly the pilot projects. To inform the mainstreaming process in an atmosphere of increased collaborative working, we identified the benefits to individuals, the health authority and the local authority.

The importance of this service to individuals was evident from the number of people who accessed the service. The increasing number of individuals accessing the service demonstrated a gap in existing alternative methods of delivering benefits advice. The evaluation demonstrated that benefits advice in primary care increased the incomes of individuals who for various reasons depended on this income. Individuals interviewed as part of this study who have made successful claims reported less worrying, less stress and increased wellbeing. Some of the elderly people interviewed identified 'being able to buy a wheelchair', 'keeping the heating on in winter' and 'eating more healthy food' as a result of receiving Attendance Allowance.

In this evaluation, we gathered many case studies, stories and anecdotes of improvements in health and wellbeing. GP practices that already host the services reported that, even though the number of consultations initially increased as the projects developed, the number of inappropriate consultations actually decreased, enabling GPs to concentrate on services they are trained to offer. Clearly benefits to the health of individuals and a decreased number of inappropriate GP consultations are beneficial to the health authority.

Local authorities not only have a statutory responsibility for providing welfare rights services but it was clear they had a tradition of supporting the community in doing this kind of work. In Camden in particular we identified a range of organisations doing income-maximisation work. The HAZ projects learnt from and linked to a number of projects, such as the income maximisation work of the Caversham Practice and targeted work, such as the CAB's housebound project and the Irish Elders project. Another reason for local authorities to provide, support and enhance benefits advice services is that the government grant aid to local authorities under the Standard Spending Assessment takes into account indicators derived from benefits take-up, including all of the live Attendance Allowance claims (Islington Welfare Rights Unit, 2001).

Conclusion

The projects were found to be successful to varying degrees, attributable to management factors, particularly the capacity of service providers, and contextual factors, in particular the circumstances among GP practices. These evaluations demonstrated a gap in service delivery and a significant need for benefits advice services. Benefits advice in primary care clearly improved people's incomes and improved their wellbeing. Clients' annual incomes clearly and significantly improved. While there were some obstacles to providing benefits advice services in primary care, these obstacles could be easily overcome. In contrast, obstacles faced by individuals to claiming benefits were far greater. This study concluded that providing benefits advice services in primary care, in particular from GP practices with targeted outreach work and home visits, clearly reduces obstacles to claiming, improves access to advice and benefits, improves incomes, and contributes to the health and wellbeing of Camden and Islington residents.

References

Acheson, D. (chair) (1998) *Independent inquiry into inequalities in health report*, London: The Stationery Office.

Camden and Islington Health Authority (2001) *Public health annual report*, London: Camden and Islington Health Authority.

Costigan, P., Finch, H., Jackson, B., Legard, R. and Richie, J. (1999) *Overcoming barriers: older people and income support*, DSS Research Report 100, Leeds: Corporate Document Services.

Islington Welfare Rights Unit (2001) *Rights: welfare rights in Islington. Income maximisation, 2001/2001*, Islington.

CHAPTER 19

The Pampering Gang Project

Dr Sohail Bhatti, Veronica Cuthbert and Jane Lunt

Summary

Caring for young children in disadvantaged circumstances carries with it an increased risk of poor maternal mental health. Interventions that enhance psychosocial support are seen to benefit maternal health. A pilot 'Pampering Day' (organised by health visitors in response to requests from mothers for postnatal support) provided aromatherapy, beauty treatments and healthy lifestyle advice – and as a result initially was awarded £10,000 HAZ monies and made sustainable by a further £7000 a year later. This chapter traces the development, planning, delivery and evolution of the project, which now offers weekly drop-in sessions, free of charge. There are successful working partnerships with a local community organisation, which provides premises; a further education college, which supplies student hairdressers and beauticians; and a local childcare charity, which supplies crèche facilities; health visitors and midwives also participate in the sessions. Until recently the initiative was overseen by a steering group, one-third being local mothers, but following an inaugural general meeting a board of management was elected, two-thirds of whom are local mothers. The Pampering Gang has now become 'owned' by the local mothers, duly empowered by the original initiative.

Context

A group of four health visitors (HVs) who worked in an area of high deprivation in Wirral (Tranmere, Birkenhead), with a significant number of isolated women with young children, often with complex health and social needs, recognised that the HV and other services were being poorly used. Historically, service provision had proved difficult because of poor attendance, especially by those in highest need. This is a common professional issue. It is being addressed nationally through the development of the public health role of both the health visitor and school nurse (DoH, 2001). Training resource packs are to be supplied to every practitioner to help challenge the traditional child development model that HVs practice, without much supporting evidence (Hall, 2000). This traditional model of postnatal groups in Wirral meant weekly sessions over a six-week time span offered in a health setting (clinic or hospital based). The content of these sessions was designed by the professionals themselves, and usually took the form of a group led by the HV. Topics covered included feeding, sleep management, minor ailments, and baby resuscitation, as well as postnatal physical and emotional wellbeing. The sixth and final session was for mothers to choose their own topic.

The content and quality of this programme varied. At that time there was no external assessment or validation, though such a tool, People into Parents ('PIPs'), was being piloted locally, but poor attendance of the postnatal support programme meant it had limited success. That these sessions were inappropriate and inaccessible was demonstrated by the poor attendance and perseverance of participants, particularly by those who had the greatest needs as a result of their poverty and isolation, as well as poor self-esteem (Acheson, 1998).

Local factors

The challenge for HVs in trying to explore new ways of working was in the heavy caseload (typically 255 families per HV) living in an area of deprivation: much time was inevitably spent on complex issues such as child protection and domestic violence – Tranmere ranks 58th out of 8414 wards in England in terms of its deprivation (DETR, 2000). Via a service level agreement with Wirral Health Authority, 10% of HV time was allocated locally for 'public health work'. This enabled the HVs to approach this issue through their hypothecated 'public health time', and thereby minimise the risk to the existing structure and professional practices. Between themselves they developed the concept and how that would impact upon their work, and then used their 'public health time' to pilot the project.

There was also the added advantage of Wirral's being part of the largest Health Action Zone in England: Merseyside. The HAZ in Merseyside has four overall goals:

1. to reduce levels of poor health, through modernising and improving health and social care services
2. to promote healthy employment opportunities
3. to increase the proportion of people who have an active independent life
4. to enhance people's quality of life. (Merseyside HAZ, 1999)

It was becoming clear that the project would contribute, albeit in a small way, to two of these overall goals (1 and 4) in the effort to change health culture in the primary care setting.

Community involvement is also one of the guiding principles of Health Action Zones, and is defined as 'A range of practices dedicated to increasing the strength and effectiveness of community life, improving local conditions, especially for people in disadvantaged situations, and enabling people to participate in public decision-making processes and to achieve greater long term control over their circumstances' (Community Development Foundation, cited in Merseyside HAZ, 2001, 8).

The aims of the project were:

- to improve the confidence and self-esteem of mothers with young children
- to build social networks and peer-group support for vulnerable families
- to reduce mental illness in the target group
- to reduce dependence on GPs in their mentoring/pastoral roles
- to improve access to and knowledge of health care/social support services
- to improve knowledge of and attitudes to behaviours beneficial to health
- to provide a forum where a hard-to-reach client group can be consulted.

Starting off

Listening to clients' views and their expressed needs

It was recognised by the HVs at the outset that they were revisiting previous HV philosophy and practice: listen to what the client has to say about what she wants, and then act upon it. Listening, according to Ledwith (1997), means you 'receive the message that you are worthy of being heard', a process vital for human functioning and one crucial to the ultimate aim of an HV: helping those children whose mothers struggle to bring them up, against all the odds. With better attendance for postnatal advice and higher self-esteem in their mothers, these children can expect a surer start in life.

Informal contact with some mothers within the target area led to the development of a service which was tailored to attracting these specific groups. By listening to and seeking opinions from these mothers, it was determined that getting personal care and attention through grooming and 'being pampered' was important to them. This was externally validated by the observation that those who can afford it spend considerable sums on personal grooming and beauty treatments to enhance their sense of wellbeing.

Public health time of HVs

The HVs involved believed that looking beyond the practice of one-to-one consultations and home visiting was the key issue. They saw the HV role as working with others to enable the community as a whole to increase its control over the determinants of health (Anderson, 1993, cited in Russell, 1999). From this understanding an empowerment model of working developed, i.e. interventions that raised people's consciousness about issues, developed their skills and understanding of situations, and encouraged self-assertiveness (WHO, 1986).

The Pilot

A venue was needed that could accommodate a number of women and children, and also lend itself to a range of people providing various 'beauty treatments'. The environment ought to offer privacy and a sense of calm and relaxation, as well as somewhere for people to gather, share a cup of tea and talk, and yet be safe for children. A steering group was convened which endorsed the decision to offer non-complex treatments that could be delivered quickly, and to offer the session to women with children under five years of age in the Lairdside area (a redevelopment area within Tranmere). The age limit complied with existing professional boundaries, as the HV service on Wirral then limited itself to families with children under five years of age. Two women that were clients were recruited to the steering group, and subsequently provided hospitality and a reception service.

Resources

A local GP offered the use of his outreach Teenage Advisory Clinic (in a multistorey block of flats), and Health Links, the local health promotion service situated within the community trust, provided (free of charge) the two aromatherapists/beauticians. Friends, colleagues and the local chemist provided a range of toiletries, and beverages were supplied by the HVs. The team spirit was strongly bolstered by the sense of trying something innovative and even daring. It was a vital component to the successful outcome of the day, as was the fact that the team included not only the HV colleagues but also local mothers involved in the session.

Beneficiaries/clients

Twelve women and their children attended the pilot session. The maternal age range varied from 18 to 42 years. The children's ages ranged from 6 weeks to 4 years. Of the women who attended, two did not regularly access the HV service and were considered 'hard to reach'. This attendance reflected the short advertising span and poor publicity (lasting only 10 days). Feedback highlighted that they all 'wanted to be there', that it was fun and that clients wanted more. The need for a crèche facility was identified, as time-out from their children was a major factor in helping women to relax and feel 'pampered'. The venue was not a popular choice as it was in a building which at that time had a negative profile within the community. There were other issues which needed to be addressed, such as severe ethical concerns. After heated debate it was agreed that by utilising insured, qualified and accredited holistic and beauty therapists, and by observing the UKCC Code of Professional Conduct (UKCC, 1992) the pilot could be developed into a service that minimised the risks of coercion and promoted informed consent.

Engaging allies

It was felt that the steering group needed to broaden its representation, and make allies. An informal approach was made to the director of public health, advising her of the pilot and the positive responses from the mothers. Her reaction was encouraging and supportive, and the HVs were advised to see the consultant for public health aligned with Birkenhead. On hearing of the initiative, he (Dr Sohail Bhatti) immediately recognised the value of what was being attempted, and volunteered his services to the steering group. A bid for funds was then developed and submitted to the Birkenhead Primary Care Group (PCG), which had received an allocation of Merseyside HAZ funding. The bid of £10,000 HAZ monies was awarded in its entirety for the 'Pampering Gang' as a pilot service.

Writing the bid made explicit the project's aim to reach mothers who did not access the health visiting or other services. One perspective from the PCG was that the project might be an alternative ('social Prozac') to traditional treatments for postnatal depression, such as antidepressants, and might also reduce prescribing cost pressures. Also, as well as being non-labelling and non-stigmatising, it was intervention that the women genuinely welcomed. The innovative nature of the approach required credible academic evaluation, so arrangements were then made for Liverpool John Moores University (Liverpool JMU) to administer the finance under the auspices of a research project.

Partnership working

As it was necessary to acquire an alternative venue at nil or minimal cost, the steering group made links with and engaged other agencies. A local community agency (Tranmere Alliance) offered the free use of their community hall for one day per week, but following a risk assessment this was deemed unsuitable. In true partnership spirit the local housing manager facilitated free use of a Residents Association flat in a tower block, so the service began approximately one year after the initial pilot.

The beneficial effect of this assistance was that the steering group expanded its membership to reflect the contribution from different partners and agencies. A local children's charity, CHUC (Committed to Helping & Understanding Children), an HV manager, the local housing manager and, most importantly, a number of women who 'sampled' the pilot became involved. The mothers who attended were not penalised financially as any expenses they had accrued for childcare were met through the budget.

Resources and further funding

The head of the hair and beauty department at the local college was contacted, and embraced the concept of the Pampering Gang. She immediately agreed to provide students, with their tutor, on a weekly placement to offer treatments. This enabled her to meet a number of her objectives, such as a community setting for her student training and potential new students from those who received such treatments. This partnership has worked well up to the present day and continues – some students have committed to provide the service outside of the college year in their own time, and are paid appropriate expenses.

One holistic therapist provided aromatherapy, baby massage, reflexology and other treatments, allowing her to develop relationships of mutual trust with the women. CHUC provided their mobile crèche facility and provided a safe, stimulating environment for children while mothers were 'pampered'. Thus children were also benefiting from the Pampering Gang activities by accessing good quality childcare. Owing to increasing awareness and interest in the project, and the ensuing lack of space in the ground-floor flat, the mobile crèche team were obliged to withdraw their services for safety reasons. This brought about a temporary halt to the activities until more suitable premises were sought. The local community hall owned by Tranmere Alliance (the original planned venue) was due to be refurbished, so it appeared that the delay would only be a few months.

The local housing manager then provided a large self-contained lounge with attached kitchen in another high-rise block of flats close to a local primary school. This allowed the sessions to resume until the community hall reopened. As there was not enough space for the mobile crèche in the new flat,7 the children were minded by their mothers, with others contributing to storybook reading, nursery rhymes and play. At the monthly steering group meetings one third of the members were now the local mothers.

On International Women's Day, six months after the project began, the Pampering Gang took part in a display of local initiatives provided by women for women. At this time further funding of £7000 had been procured by the project from the Public Health New Initiatives Fund, providing the project with a healthy bank balance and increased optimism for seeking future funding. This was opportunistic, but reflected the developmental nature of the project as three of the original four HVs were now seconded to public health in a new role as outreach/community facilitators: public health facilitators.

Outcomes and evaluation

Improved access to services for the target population

Tranmere Alliance gained further funds for refurbishment from a variety of sources, including an award of HAZ monies, the project having increased local awareness of the need for the upgrading. In order to comply with regulations, and as an example of the momentum gathering around the Pampering Gang, a separate area was created which would meet the criteria set by childcare regulations.

Improved social networks for the community members: family events

At the steering group meetings the mothers proposed various suggestions regarding specific activities and events. The first event was the Children's Easter party, held on the premises of a Community Development Trust, which incorporated elements of the Take 5 Healthy Eating Programme, a benefit in health terms that cannot be overstated. Other suggestions taken up included a funded visit by coach to a children's theme park, and to accommodate a holiday play scheme a return visit was made to the previous venue for a teddy bears' picnic.

Improved understanding of the needs of this population

A certain intimacy has developed within the Pampering Gang. This results from women attending for varying periods of time beginning to feel safe, secure and among 'friends'. Women then divulge information that they may not have told anyone else: the response they get from the other women in terms of help, support and empathy is the intangible extra which builds confidence and self-esteem, and empowers lonely people, making them into networks of friends, not strangers. This intimacy, perceived by both the mothers and the HVs, acts as an interface which eases mutual exchange of information in a confidential and comfortable environment, and leads to increased mutual awareness and appreciation.

Future commissioning of targeted outreach by PCGs/PCTs

As a result of anecdotal feedback from mothers and HVs, together with the recognition within the fourth-wave Sure Start (the Ferries Programme based in Tranmere) of the benefits of the Pampering Gang model, there is an increased awareness of the project among local GPs in the PCG who are supportive of this particular approach. It is intended following the formal evaluation that the results will be published and presented to the PCG/T for consideration for commissioning and expansion, if so desired by mothers in adjacent areas.

Evaluation with Liverpool JMU: structured questionnaires on self-esteem and wellbeing

Evaluation is about judging the worth of an activity (Peberdy, 1999). The activities undertaken at the Pampering Gang were designed to increase self-esteem and confidence in the mothers, encourage increased knowledge of and attitudes to behaviours beneficial to health, and reduce mental illness. It was also hoped to demonstrate that these achievements constituted an empowering process. These are all nebulous and contested concepts (Peberdy, 1999). Approaches and links were made with Liverpool JMU, and an individual with an interest in this field joined the steering group. A screening questionnaire was devised to be administered when women joined the group to obtain baseline information on their perceived self-esteem, confidence, support networks and their current mental wellbeing. This questionnaire would then be repeated after a period of time (the suggested time span was 10–12 weeks), and any perceived change in these determinants would be observed. In parallel with this formal consultative evaluation there was also the process of participatory evaluation determined by the mothers involved with the project. The initial questionnaire was modified following a pilot run, but owing to the fact that the full service of the Pampering Gang included crèche facilities which were not available until transfer into refurbished premises in late summer 2001, the process of evaluation has of necessity been subject to delay.

Powerful written comments and photographs have been produced that have been used at events (including the HAZ Conference at Wakefield, September 2001) to demonstrate the benefits to these women. A founder member of the Pampering Gang (Veronica Cuthbert) is currently undertaking doctoral studies which will explore issues of empowerment of mothers arising from the project.

Sustainability

Negotiations took place with Liverpool JMU for transfer of funds to a community bank account in order that the long-term aims of the project, i.e. ownership of the group by local mothers, could be progressed. Consultation with increasing numbers of mothers attending the weekly sessions indicated their support towards establishing their own constitution, so providing the opportunity for the creation of a board of management. Members agreed an agenda for an inaugural general meeting, on Halloween 2001, which gave the opportunity for a party as well as a memorable date for successive AGMs. Poster and flyers were produced and circulated via local health visitors and steering group members. Expressions of interest had been received from the mothers to take on roles within the board, and each officer post had at least one name nominated. On the day, about 40 people attended (plus children). There was a party lunch after which the draft constitution was accepted (with minor amendments) followed by election of the chair and other officers of the board of management. The chair and vice-chair, secretary and four committee members were local mothers, and the elected treasurer was the community worker from the local Community Development Trust, while the two remaining board members elected were local health visitors. The current project leader and chair of the steering group was co-opted as adviser to assist with capacity building of the newly elected board.

Ownership by local mothers

It was always envisaged by the HVs that the control and future of the group lay with the women involved, and that ultimately the HVs' role would change to providing a presence in a health advisory capacity. This would guarantee the continuance of the group and would come about as a direct result of the women feeling empowered to take control of the group. On the day of their election both chair and vice-chair spoke enthusiastically of their intention to continue consultation with local mothers, and to make their views and choices known. Handover arrangements were planned with the project manager, so ensuring ongoing support and capacity building for this newly emerging and exciting community initiative.

Capacity building

This is recognised as a vital process in the development of any project, and as such has been recognised by group members. Approaches have been made to the local Council for Voluntary Service (Wirral CVS) for provision initially of a bespoke programme to undertake a team-building day with appropriate timings, venue and crèche to facilitate the participation of members who have family commitments. This organisation also provides an ongoing development programme throughout the year which is accessible by all voluntary groups dealing with the acquisition of skills (e.g. minute taking) or updating of information.

Funding opportunities

A well-recognised requirement by current funders is for groups to be formally established and accountable with appropriate methods for audit trail. The Pampering Gang meets such requirements, and having had early success with funding is in a position to make application for further funding from a variety of local initiatives, including the fourth-wave Sure Start Programme, the local council, the primary care group and local charities.

Sure Start Programme

Currently, a fourth-wave Sure Start in the Rock Ferry/Tranmere area has adopted the model to use in the Sure Start bases, acknowledging that to engage isolated and hard-to-reach mothers an alternative approach to traditional methods needs to be taken. Reaching this group is integral to the Sure Start programme (www.surestart.gov.uk). As word has spread both locally and further afield, requests for further information and visits have been arranged in consultation with the mothers. A call and follow-up visit from a Sure Start Programme in a nearby authority has resulted in their adoption of the model, and strong links have been formed between the two groups.

Conclusions

As a result of the initiative, the project since inception has had in excess of 1000 contacts for a cost of £8000 in human and financial resource (less of the latter), and has still £12,000 in the bank, at a consumption rate of £5000 per annum. Lessons have been learnt at every stage, and the learning and enthusiasm within and without the initiative continue to snowball among other groups and individuals. The Pampering Gang model is transferable to all age groups and genders (because it deals with the universal human need for attention and feeling valued – 'pampering'), and has been seen to bring about changes in both attitudes and practice, though not without challenge. An interesting side effect of the media publicity (e.g. newspaper articles, radio interviews) was the envy it created in members of the wider community. There was concern that at a time when waiting lists were expanding, money was being wasted on what some people regarded as 'spongers'.

However, such challenges are there to be met if inequalities and social exclusion are to be tackled within our communities. Three years after its inception, the Pampering Gang now has the strength from congruence with government policy and professional aspiration that enables it to make itself heard and understood.

Key lessons learnt

The project has shown that:

- community development approaches do work, but they take time and much effort
- refocusing of services is necessary
- successful initiatives quickly accumulate statutory sector allies, as government policy encourages all agencies to target the 'hard to reach'
- stakeholder involvement is important, as is identifying local champions
- it is important to value the team approach
- evaluation is an ethical duty
- value for money means cost effectiveness
- alliances and partnerships are vital to success.

Acknowledgement

We would like to thank, on behalf of the mothers, all the many people and agencies who are too numerous to mention but who have generously helped to make this project successful.

References

Acheson, D. (1998) *Independent enquiry into inequalities in health report,* London: Stationery Office.

DETR (2000) *Index of multiple deprivation, 2000,* London: Department of the Environment, Transport and the Regions.

DoH (2001) *Health visitor practice development resource pack,* London: Department of Health.

Hall, D. M. B. (2000) *Health for all children: joint working party report,* 3rd edn, Oxford: Oxford University Press.

Ledwith, M. (1997) *Participating in transformation: towards a working model of community empowerment,* Birmingham: Venture Press.

Merseyside HAZ (1999) *Merseyside Health Action Zone implementation plan,* Liverpool: Merseyside HAZ.

Merseyside HAZ (2001) *A step by step guide to community involvement for organisations: how well are we doing?,* Liverpool: Merseyside HAZ.

Peberdy, A. (1999) 'Evaluating community action', in: Jones, L. and Sidell, M. (eds) *The challenge of promoting health: exploration and action,* Basingstoke: Macmillan in association with The Open University.

Russell, J. (1999) 'The potential for promoting health with local communities: general practice and the primary health care team', in: Jones, L. and Sidell, M. (eds) *The challenge of promoting health: exploration and action*, Basingstoke: Macmillan in association with The Open University.

UKCC (1992) *Code of professional conduct*, London: United Kingdom Central Council for Nursing, Midwifery & Health Visiting.

WHO (1986) *Ottawa charter for health promotion*, Geneva: World Health Organization.

CHAPTER 20

Stepping out: enabling people with disabilities to participate in community leisure activities

Brigid Kane

The problem

The South Yorkshire Coalfields HAZ was set up to reduce health inequalities and to improve health, in its widest sense: 'a state of complete physical, mental and social well-being and not merely the absence of disease or infirmity' (WHO, 1948). One of the HAZ's main aims is to 'enable people with physical and sensory disabilities in later life to live more independent lives'.

There is considerable research evidence of the positive effects of physical activity on a variety of disabling conditions – not only in tackling symptoms such as pain and breathlessness, but also in improving overall mobility and physical fitness, pain control, and mental and physical wellbeing. Using community sports and leisure facilities also helps to integrate people with disabilities into society, reducing isolation and stigmatisation, which can adversely affect their quality of life.

However, people with physical and sensory disabilities have difficulty in accessing community sports and leisure facilities. These difficulties may include:

- nonexistent, or inaccessible, transport to facilities
- poor physical access to buildings
- lack of necessary equipment
- inadequate training of staff, and low awareness of disability issues
- lack of personal assistance.

Even where facilities are accessible, some people with disabilities may lack the confidence to utilise them without personal support: 'Before coming to Stepping Out I was just sat on my own, did not mix with people and had no confidence'.

Inability to access community sports and leisure facilities can have a number of negative consequences for people with physical and sensory disabilities, they may:

- become isolated and housebound
- feel 'ghetto-ised' in day care centres
- fail to improve, or exacerbate, their physical condition by not taking appropriate exercise
- develop, or worsen, mental health problems such as anxiety and depression.

Background

The South Yorkshire Coalfields is made up of three metropolitan boroughs – Barnsley, Doncaster and Rotherham. All three have suffered the economic and social consequences of the collapse of the mining and, to some extent, steel industries, on which the local economy depended. In 1981, there were 39 pits in the area – by the early 1990s this had been reduced to 4. Ex-miners form a cohort of men now predominantly aged over 50, with high levels of long-term limiting illness and a high take-up of incapacity benefit. Women are also suffering, both from the adverse effects of the industrial past and the present effects of low employment and loss of social cohesion. In a recent study of nine local communities (Green et al., 2000), the level of limiting long-term illness found in the coalfield communities was significantly higher than the British average – see Figure 20.1. Stepping Out was established as a pilot project in Barnsley in 1999, at the request of disabled people who wanted a more holistic and socially inclusive alternative to traditional day care and hospital-based rehabilitation programmes. They wanted 'to have a life, not just a care package'.

The advent of the SYC HAZ enabled the service to be a expanded to cover all three boroughs: this paper is largely based on a project evaluation carried out in 2001 by Sue Ryder Care at the end of its first full year of activity.

The aim of Stepping Out is to engage disabled people in ordinary leisure and sports activities within the wider community, to provide both health and social outcomes. It not only offers a wide variety of activities, but also breaks down the barriers to participation by tackling transport, access and personal care issues.

Approach

Stepping Out is managed by a voluntary organisation, Sue Ryder Care. It recruited four staff (2.3 full-time equivalents) and provided them with an extensive training programme and the use of a minibus. Training courses undertaken by staff included:

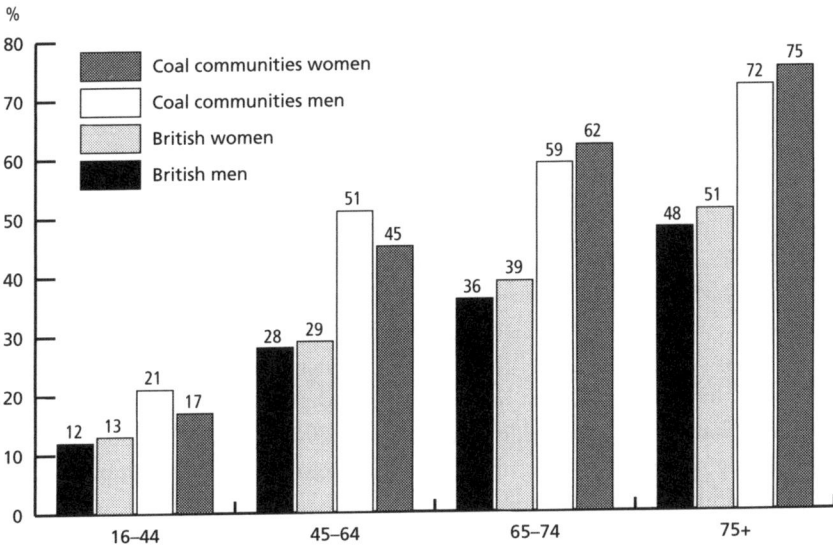

Source: Office for National Statistics (1998), *General household survey*, table 7.1.

Figure 20.1: Percentage with limiting long-term illness by age group

- NVQ Care Level 2
- NVQ Assessors Award
- disability equality
- first aid
- care of medicine
- health and safety
- moving and handling
- minibus safety
- counselling
- courses on epilepsy, Huntington's disease, spina bifida, cystic fibrosis, multiple sclerosis and Parkinson's disease
- making and editing a video (for producing participants' video diaries).

Self-referrals (23%) and those from voluntary organisations (10%) were accepted, although the majority of referrals came from social services (39%) and therapists (28%).

Following referral, a Stepping Out manager will contact the individual to carry out a home visit and assessment. From the assessment, the Stepping Out manager will work with the client to draw up an action plan, which sets out their social and health goals. This document also informs the rest of the team of any care needs the individual may have and the safest way to meet these needs. Once the individual starts with the group, observations and daily records will be made on each activity undertaken, with a review after three months to check the placement is suitable. After this, the individual will be allocated to a key worker, and every eight weeks they will meet to discuss any problems, issues, achievements or outcomes. The project operates on three days a week and each client participates, on average, in two activities on one day per week, with additional social events for the whole of the current group.

Every three months, staff produce a report giving information on what the individual has participated in, how often, and what health and social wellbeing outcomes have been achieved. Stepping Out staff always seek to engage clients in assessing their own needs throughout the programme. For example, in one three-monthly review, one team member reported:

> Her health has deteriorated slightly and she finds it increasingly difficult to carry on doing a full day of physical exercise and then go home and look after her teenage son. She has talked this over with staff and it was suggested that she alternates her exercise, e.g. swim one week and gym the next, then for the rest of the day do light activities such as bowls or skittles. The client was in full agreement and is finding she does not feel as tired when she gets home, and feels a lot better about herself.

The range of conditions encountered in clients to date was extremely varied, with the largest numbers having head or spinal injury, multiple sclerosis, epilepsy and arthritis, and a further 14 conditions covered by the 'other' category (see Figure 20.2).

A total of 36 people participated in the project in its first full year, with a waiting list of 20 by the end of the year. The project worked in partnership with a variety of statutory and voluntary organisations, and with the principal leisure centre in each district, to offer a wide range of activities. The types of activities offered, and the number participating in each, is shown in Table 20.1.

The evaluation of the project has been based upon the following material:

- progress to desired outcomes for individuals
- measures of social capital, for example levels of trust and self-respect, self-reported by clients at regular meetings with staff
- general health measures, self-reported by clients
- video diaries (a brief overview video is available)
- quantitative data from project records

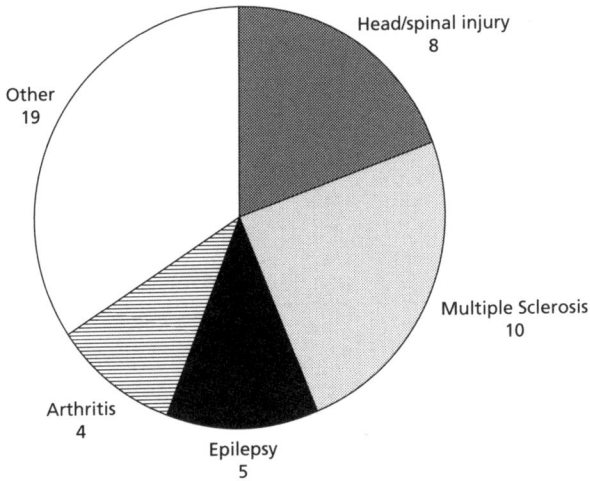

Note: Some participants have more than one condition.

Figure 20.2: Participants' medical conditions

Table 20.1 Physical and leisure activities offered

Physical activities	Participants	Leisure activities	Participants
Swimming	36	Museums	34
Bowling	19	Coast	35
Skittles	17	Parks	34
Badminton	9	Garden centres	35
Gym	36	Shopping/factory outlets	35
Relaxation therapy	36	Evening pursuits	34
Ice skating	4	Social events	36
Aromatherapy	15		
Board games	10		
Air hockey	6		
Sunbed	1		

- qualitative reports by Stepping Out manager
- case studies, approved by the individuals concerned
- material from Dr C. Dowzer et al., *Living with multiple health conditions: a systematic search and literature review*, 1999 (a report for the American Association of Retired Persons).

Table 20.2 Percentage of participants reporting health and social benefits

Health benefits	%	Social benefits	%
Improved psychological wellbeing	69	Enabled participation in community activities	100
Improved physical wellbeing	89	Improved choice in day care	44
Improved circulation in limbs	47	Reduced isolation and loneliness	83
Improved respiration	11	Increased feelings of self-worth	100
Improved mobility	39	New friendships	100
More flexibility of joints	39	Return to ordinary family activities	31
Prevention of additional illnesses		Learning new hobbies	67
and disabilities	19	Return to work	6

Outcomes and lessons learnt

Overall positive outcomes were reported by a high proportion of the participants, in terms of both health and social wellbeing. Table 20.2 gives the percentage of participants reporting each type of benefit.

Some of the participants' comments, recorded on the project video (made with the support of Northern College), summarise the change the project has made to their lives:

- 'My balance has improved since coming to Stepping Out, as well as my walking. Getting into the water and being able to get out of my chair – it is fantastic!'
- 'For the first time in five years, I go into a big supermarket by myself. I can pick and choose. I do not have to rely on others. Coming to Stepping Out has changed my life around.'
- 'I want to be like anyone else ... out enjoying myself.'
- 'There are so many choices put to us, both individually and as a group. I have been to so many places ... I just feel like a human being again.'

The case study shown in Box 20.1 is one of many examples of the significant changes the project has made to the physical and social wellbeing of its participants.

A number of valuable outcomes were also identified for the health and social care system, including:

- reduced pressure on day care centres
- increased alternatives for social services/therapy services
- improved outcomes compared to medical rehabilitation alone
- developing partnerships with individuals and voluntary sector agencies
- over 50 training courses completed by project staff
- improved awareness of staff and accessibility of main sports centres in each district.

Box 20.1 Case study: Chris

Chris was a 25-year-old professional footballer when he was severely injured in a road traffic accident. He sustained severe brain injuries, leaving him with no balance or mobility, affecting his vision and speech, and causing him to have mood swings. Chris's family heard about the Stepping Out project through a friend and realised it could help him to rediscover his interest in exercise.

When he first started to attend group swimming sessions, Chris could only swim in circles and relied heavily on a float around his body and neck. Walking in water has improved his balance and coordination and he can now walk with a tripod frame. He has many new friends and his mood swings are now less dramatic. His improvement has been sufficient that his family were able to take him on holiday and he could swim with them, using a float borrowed from the project.

His father said 'Chris really enjoyed the physical side of the activities. Now that he has finished the programme, we will carry on. I go to the gym with him and we do the same kind of things that he learnt from Stepping Out.'

The project also learnt some important lessons:

- Transport is a major problem. Up to 25% of project time was taken up in collecting participants in the minibus from across the three boroughs, which was resented by the participants. Participants who were ready to move on from the project were often deterred from continuing to utilise sports and leisure facilities by both the costs and access problems of public transport and the perceived inflexibility of community transport.

- The project had unexpected benefits for economic regeneration. The increased self-esteem generated by participation in the project encouraged some people into education or training, and two found employment.

- The scale of the project was inadequate to meet demand. There was a waiting list of 20 by the end of the first full year of operation, in which 36 people participated.

- More administration time was needed to provide adequate reports and undertake evaluations with participants. The scale of the project allowed only 12.5% of staff time to be spent on administration.

- Inadequate physical access to some facilities limited the availability of activities. The project therefore sees a need to lobby for improved accessibility.

Implications for policy and practice

Stepping Out has taken an innovative approach to improving the health and wellbeing of people with physical and sensory disabilities. Generally, clinicians and policy makers rely on objective measures to plan services, such as limitations in activities of daily living, or hospital readmission rates, and tend to focus provision on a medical model of physical and mental rehabilitation. This approach, however, fails to recognise the improvements that can be made in patients' quality of life by combining physical activity with patient-centred decision making (including self-referral) and social rehabilitation, through integration into a wide range of ordinary community physical and leisure activities.

The participants in the first full year of this project have demonstrated positive effects on their physical and mental wellbeing (as opposed to simply reduction of illness or symptoms), which have resulted in reduced demand for NHS and social care services, and increased independence. The responses to the project of therapists who were initially sceptical are worth noting:

- 'No-one we have referred to Stepping Out has returned to our service. Some clients had been with us for a number of years and we are aware of their progress.'
- 'I felt Sue Ryder was wrong in promoting resources being used in the community, that outcomes could not be achieved. I now have to re-think given the evidence I see'.

Furthermore, this improved quality of life has been achieved at a relatively low cost of £41,100 per annum, or £1142 per participant per year. There is a challenge to policy makers and service planners, however, to review their current models of service provision and dedicate funding to this innovative social model of rehabilitation.

In addition to mainstream funding, there are a number of other areas in which improvements will be needed if the success of this project is to be built on and replicated elsewhere, including:

- Those involved in planning regeneration strategies, and initiatives such as Welfare to Work, should take note of the effectiveness of this form of rehabilitation in enabling people with disabilities to access education, training and employment, and build it into their support programmes.
- Statutory, voluntary and private sector providers of leisure and sports facilities should ensure that their services are accessible to people with disabilities, and their staff appropriately trained, so as to meet the spirit, as well as the letter, of the Disability Discrimination Act 1995.

- Improvements are needed to the availability and accessibility of transport, to enable people with disabilities to access community sports and leisure provision: the current Social Exclusion Unit consultation on transport and social exclusion may assist in this.

Overall, Stepping Out has demonstrated that it offers an effective approach to enabling people with physical or sensory disabilities (congenital or acquired) to live more independently, maximise their physical health and mobility, reach their full potential and participate in community life – all of which are objectives of the South Yorkshire Coalfields HAZ.

Acknowledgement

This paper is based on an unpublished evaluation report produced by the project development manager in the summer of 2001.

References

Green, G., Grimley, M., Suokas, A., Prescott, M., Jowitt, T., Linacre, R. (2000) *Social capital, health and economy in South Yorkshire coalfield communities*, Sheffield Hallam University, Centre for Regional Economic and Social Research.

WHO (1948) 'Preamble to the constitution of the World Health Organization as adopted by the International Health Conference, New York, 19–22 June 1946', *Official Records of the World Health Organization*, 2, 100 [available at http://www.who.int/m/topicgroups/who_organization/en/].

CHAPTER 21

Addressing inequalities in health: education and training as a catalyst for change and innovation

Liz Rodrigo and Rachel Munton

Introduction

This chapter will outline the ways in which education and training, broadly defined, have been prioritised across all Leicester HAZ workstreams as a way of addressing inequalities in health. It will describe the steps that have been taken to outline and focus the agenda, and the development and operationalisation of a strategic framework, and the way in which this framework has been widely disseminated and used to underpin professionally robust, transparent protocols. Specific examples of the workstreams' activities will illustrate the ways in which education and training can be used as a catalyst for change and innovation. Particular emphasis will be placed on the ways in which these activities both reflect and shape the modernisation agenda. This chapter will introduce this strategic framework ('The Six Is'), and show how it has been operationalised.

Sustainable change and evaluation protocols will be discussed, and the chapter will conclude with a summary of lessons learnt, and the way forward.

Background

Leicester City Health Action Zone encompasses the entire city of Leicester, population 324,473 (OPCS, 1991), a richly ethnically diverse city where 80% of people in some wards are of Asian subcontinent origin. There are many wards with profound and longstanding deprivation: 13 of the 28 wards in the city fall within the most deprived 10% nationally, and a further 6 in the most deprived 11–20% (Leicestershire Health Authority, 2001).

Leicester HAZ is fortunate to have within its area one city council and two primary care trusts. There are two universities that work collaboratively through the Health Action Zone and provide postgraduate and undergraduate training. Historically Leicester has been dependent on the textile industry for employment.

The role of education and training

The Leicester Health Action Zone has been innovative by prioritising education and training as a means of addressing inequalities in health. As a discrete workstream with a small, dedicated team, education and training activities are ideally placed to contribute to the wider HAZ agenda, all of which reflects national and local priorities. Built on a reputation for educational expertise, the team have been consulted at regional level in relation to recruitment and retention, development of education for Patient Advocacy Liaison Service (PALS) Pathfinder sites and rollout of PALS initiatives.

However, the breadth of the potential agenda has required the identification of a strategic framework that delineates the distinguishing and differentiating features of HAZ educational activities. A lack of clarity about HAZ activities locally made this framework an essential early goal. Three core strands of activity have been identified under the broad headings of workforce development, inter-agency and interdisciplinary activities, and the support and funding of education and training programmes.

The activities of the education and training subcommittee support this agenda. A small but committed group of people initially took forward the education and training workstream in 1999, following the agreement for Leicester to be a second-wave Health Action Zone. Initially this subcommittee had representatives from both Leicester universities, all NHS Trusts, local social services, and the local Training and Enterprise Council (now Learning and Skills Council). One of the subcommittee's first tasks was to appoint two education and training coordinators to service their initial aims:

- to achieve in Leicester a public sector workforce better able to handle the challenges of working in the new, integrated, community-orientated NHS
- to develop a workforce capable of managing change, and ultimately creating a critical mass of workers able to positively influence service evolution to ensure service delivery matches the agenda of Leicester communities, particularly where inequalities in health are greatest.

Development of the 'Six Is' strategic framework

The coordinators developed these aims and a supporting strategic framework to guide their work and maintain the focus of the workstream, and to reflect HAZ priorities nationally and locally.

It became apparent at the start that the task ahead of the coordinators could be too immense if not firmly focused on the principles and aims of the Health Action Zone. The HAZ principles as stated in HAZnet (2001) are:

- achieving equity
- engaging communities
- working in partnership
- engaging frontline staff
- taking an evidence-based approach
- developing a person-centred approach to service delivery
- taking a whole systems approach.

For those familiar with and immersed in HAZ culture these are self-evident; however, there was a need to translate these priorities, and make them more explicit and transparent, to the diversity of partners and stakeholders, each of whom has their own priorities and agendas.

The 'Six Is' framework

This framework was developed as a tool to focus activity, add clarity and render the workstream's activities accessible to the wide audience with whom the HAZ works. A mnemonic was used deliberately to reflect the prime minister's five Ps in relation to the modernisation agenda (DoH, 2000), and to help concentrate on the workstream's proper focus.

Inequalities

Initiatives are desired to address inequalities in access, process or outcome in health and social care – for example, ameliorating coronary heart disease risk factors in minority ethnic communities – and/or in access, process and outcome of education and training for those working within health and social care – for example, workplace development, recruitment and retention.

Imperatives

Initiatives should tackle the National and Leicester HAZ priority areas:

- coronary heart disease
- cancer
- mental health
- drug abuse prevention
- waiting lists, winter pressures and service modernisation
- children and families
- minority ethnic health
- promoting positive health
- community development/capacity building.

Innovation

Ideas are wanted that are either new, creative or pilot in nature, and attract subsequent funding from elsewhere if successfully evaluated as sustainable projects.

Initiation

HAZ education and training monies are intended to initiate, to 'pump prime', and are non-recurrent. The education and training coordinators will assist successful projects in endeavours to secure subsequent funding to promote sustainability.

Involvement

Projects and activities should demonstrate the active involvement of service users, carers, and other recipients of health and social care.

Interdisciplinary

Programmes are encouraged to foster interdisciplinary and inter-agency education and training, and thus collaboration and working practice.

This strategic framework has been operationalised, informing the wide range of workstream activity. For example, it has acted as an assessment and scoring tool against which requests for funding, assessments of requests for support, and the education coordinators' activities are assessed. If the requested activity falls outside of these strategic imperatives, then referral is made to other, specified, agencies for support. There has not yet been any follow-up of how/whether those recommendations were taken up, or not, and this is the prospective focus of an externally conducted and funded evaluative research project. There is, however, anecdotal evidence that the strategic framework developed by the team, and the application of this theoretical framework to practice, has led to a clear understanding of HAZ goals and to clear service improvements. A variety of new and innovative educational programmes are currently supported; service users are actively engaged at all levels; frontline workers are engaged in high-quality, externally accredited education programmes. There are increased opportunities to experience 'tasters' in health and social care careers, and recruitment initiatives to support the development of a workforce more representative of the city's population are under way. Specific interventions, which address the future workforce needs, will illustrate the collaboration required to achieve the objectives of the human resources strategy and the imperatives of the modernisation agenda (DoH, 2000).

Educational activities as a catalyst for change

Learning from the current activities can be distilled and integrated into the changing landscape of health and social care. A focus on partnerships and shared learning with Leicester City PCTs and the emerging local strategic partnership illustrate the workstream's forward focus on sustainability. It is necessary to formally evaluate the impact of these educative activities on inequalities in health, and to focus on interventions which address the future workforce needs. In all of these activities, given the demography of Leicester City, issues of minority ethnic groups are central, and have been embraced. The following illustrates some current projects.

The projects funded are varied and show considerable potential in tackling health inequalities. Although not formally externally evaluated there is abundant evidence of practice development and partnership working in the lifetime of these projects. Brief reviews illustrate the achievements to date.

Educating mental health service users: PLUS+

With the Leicester HAZ as a catalyst, three partners joined together to develop a protocol for the education of twelve mental health service users, to an agenda that is evolved and set by them, with a view to developing their skills, competence and confidence to work with other service users, and to educate health and social care professionals in subsequent periods. This cascade approach enables the needs of service users to be realistically addressed in the training of mental health and other frontline staff (Sainsbury Centre for Mental Health, 1997).

Key features of the education are the equality of all partners, the use of adult learning strategies that enhance confidence building, proactive provision of increased emotional and psychological support required by participants exposed to such new and emotive experiences, and the accreditation of the programme by a national body. The experience and activities of PLUS+ (the name the group chose, standing for Positive+Learning+Understanding+Support) will be shared. This shows that participants' experiences have applicability to other areas, both geographically and clinically in mental health care, and are highly commensurate with the NSF for mental health (DoH, 1999).

'Connect' project APEX

APEX approached Leicester HAZ education and training coordinators with a request for support in developing the knowledge and skills of their frontline workers to improve services to unemployed ex-offenders, additionally disadvantaged by disturbed or distressing behaviours, mental illness and/or substance misuse. Staff are increasingly being expected, and wishing to, deal with such difficulties, for which they feel poorly prepared and on occasion personally vulnerable.

These clients are identified as the hardest to help, are often long-term unemployed, and often have concurrent physical and/or mental health difficulties, and/or learning difficulties.

The aims of the programme are:

1 To improve the skills and knowledge of frontline staff at APEX Leicester to improve services to unemployed ex-offenders, additionally disadvantaged by disturbed or distressing behaviours, mental illness and/or substance misuse.
2 To provide a flexible, City and Guilds accredited programme of education that will fulfil the needs of staff, delivered in a way that reflects the core principles of *The capable practitioner* (Sainsbury Centre for Mental Health, 2000).

The entire APEX staff group are involved as learners, comprising trainers, trainees, volunteers, frontline staff, and administrative, advice and guidance staff (a total of approximately 40 staff, divided into 2–3 small groups of 10–15: 40 delegates commenced July 2001 on accredited training). Some of these staff may have personal experience of the criminal justice system and/or mental illness/substance misuse.

Advocacy for Cancer Patients

The aim of this project was to provide funding for people with cancer, or their carers, to have access to the Cancer Voices Course. This course empowers service users with the skills to negotiate and advocate/articulate on behalf of other cancer patients with health service professionals. This links in well with the government's current initiative of 'the expert patient' (DoH, 2001d).

Training Project Dil workers

Project Dil is a programme aimed at reducing the incidence of coronary heart disease among the South Asian community in Leicester. This community suffers disproportionately from coronary heart disease (Balarajan, 1996). One element of Project Dil has been the training of peer educators who will work with the community. HAZ Education and Training are now working with Project Dil and Cardiac Rehabilitation to develop a module that will educate peer educators to work in a paid capacity alongside their clinical colleagues, using their expertise with the community to complement the clinical skills of health professionals. This module will be accredited and build on the education that the peer educators have received to date. It is hoped that this will improve services to the patient and change working practices in the clinical setting.

Education of workers with the Single Homelessness Initiative

Building on identified training needs, and gaps within current provision, the Health Action Zone education team was approached to work alongside the homelessness multidisciplinary teams to develop a comprehensive education and training framework. This framework acknowledges and builds upon the pilot work undertaken in mental health education (2000–01), and the training needs audit of hostel workers and other frontline staff.

The aim of the programme is to improve safe client-centred care through a systematic, flexible, progressive programme of relevant education and training for staff working in frontline services for single homeless people. The programme attracts a nationally accredited award, enables the integration of theory and practice, using a reflective learning approach based on real life issues, underpinned by identified job requirements and core competencies. The programme is flexible, participative, facilitated by experts and robustly evaluated.

Sixteen frontline workers from statutory and voluntary sectors are members of the pilot group, supported by HAZ, the local Mental Health Trust and city council.

Learning for Better Health

This project focuses on the needs of those with commonly occurring mental health problems, where a prescription for education and/or training might have attendant benefits in terms of increased self-esteem, occupation and social opportunity. It is intended to evaluate the extent to which this has a beneficial impact on health, and the extent to which health care professionals make prescriptions for such activities in two inner city areas of significant deprivation. Again, this initiative demonstrates partnership initiatives between the mainstream adult education sector, the health professionals and higher education institutions. This project is run in partnership with NIACE (National Institute of Adult Continuing Education) and is in the second year of three years' funding. Research into its efficacy is central to the project, and runs parallel to it.

Ethnic Diversity CD-ROM

As stated, Leicester is an ethnically diverse city: some primary schools have over 40 languages spoken as first languages among the children. This diversity is reflected throughout the population, and hence with the patients and clients seen within the health service. Ethnic diversity training has been inconsistent within Leicester, purchased from different providers and of varying quality. Some practitioners find it difficult to release time to attend ethnic diversity training. This project aims to provide an interactive educational resource that includes the use of multimedia graphics (video, audio and graphics). It uses the community to reflect its faith and culture via the video clips within the CD-ROM and written material, which has been developed by a host of partners and validated by a representative patient council. It is hoped to address issues of sexuality, sexual health and mental health that are often avoided within ethnicity education.

Highfields project: Insight Project

This project is specially aimed at raising the awareness of the health sector as an employer among youth and adults in the Highfields area. Although Leicester city has an ethnic minority population of 30%, and in some wards over 70% of the population are from ethnic minority communities (OPCS, 1991), this is not reflected within the health sector workforce which in the community is less than 5% (personal communication, 2001). Highfields is an area of Leicester with a large ethnic minority population. This project is based in a large community college and has two parallel streams. The youth stream aims to research the current provision of health service careers information and adapt it for this community, actively involving the young people in the college to do this. The adult stream is developing a taster to the health service course for adults; this builds on the currently offered Taster to Nursing course. One of the aims of the project is to build links between the health sector and the Community College, with a view to enhancing diversity within the health workforce.

Other core workstream activities: service-user participation

As shown above, part of the Six Is is Involvement, which is expressed within all of the funded projects to some extent. It became apparent that the education and training subcommittee was solely professionally led and therefore not representing fully the principles of the workstream's practice, which is in line with the Kennedy Report (DoH, 2001c): 'the priority for involving the public should be that their interests are embedded into all organisations and institutions concerned with quality of performance in the NHS: in other words, the public should be "on the inside" rather than represented by some body "on the outside"'.

A process of defining service-user representation within the group was begun and resulted in the appointment of two service-user representatives to the committee. Despite the early stage of their appointments it is already apparent that they are influencing the work of the committee and bringing a fresh dimension to the group.

Recruitment and retention

In addition to the nationally acknowledged recruitment and retention challenges in health and social care, following the first round of funded projects there was some evidence that the lack of staff to provide cover prevented staff already employed from attending education. It has been part of the workstream's role to look at ways of addressing recruitment and retention. This has led to many projects that link education to recruitment and retention and workforce development. Figure 21.1 illustrates this structure. Some of the projects that the workstream is involved with within this area are briefly described below.

- Primary Care Trust Workforce Development: a core group are addressing the interface between the government's varied policies to tackle workforce issues, translating them to the specific profile of Leicester City. At an early stage of development, this work has acted as a springboard for a review of continuous practice development, appraisal and individual learning accounts.

- Protected Learning Times Evaluation within a Primary Care Trust: one of the PCTs organised a monthly protected learning time whereby the whole PCT was invited to centrally held education for the afternoon. The workstream was involved in the evaluation, consultation and subsequent education strategy that has emerged from this.

- NHS Career Road Show: this event is in the early planning stages for 2002 and will hopefully use some of the work from the Insight Project (above) and the Shadowing Project (below). It is planned that a four-day road show will be taken to five different schools within the city with large numbers of ethnic minority students. The road shows are intended to inform and display the diversity of careers and employment available in the health sector. This will include the illustration of career pathways for people at all stages of their academic achievement, or for those for whom academic achievement is not possible.

- Primary Care Trust Work Shadowing Project: this project has involved both PCTs to try to develop a robust structure for people of all ages to experience the health sector as a potential employer. This falls in line with the widening of participation within the health sector. In the near future it is hoped that a pilot scheme with local schools can offer work experience within the primary care setting.

Multidisciplinary educational initiatives

Refugees and Asylum Seekers

This innovative multidisciplinary pilot course aims to reduce inequalities in health through mutual information sharing, fostering greater understanding about the health service and asylum seekers'/new refugees' own experiences. This will better equip frontline workers with the skills to address the needs of a widely diverse and under-served population within the city. This course has been developed with refugee and asylum seeker lead input and facilitation.

STIF: Sexually Transmitted Infections Foundation Course

The workstream has been approached by the secondary care sector to coordinate an accredited multidisciplinary course about sexual health for frontline primary health care providers following the *Sexual health strategy* consultation document (DoH, 2001a). This again illustrates the benefits of working across health sectors.

Sure Start

Leicester City has three Sure Start projects, and plans for more and the mainstreaming of Sure Start within the city. The education and training workstream has been approached to work with Sure Start to promote and develop the educational and employment skills of parents from within the disadvantaged areas of the city as an innovative way of both addressing inequalities for children and families.

Patient Advocacy Liaison Service (PALS)

The workstream is participating in the local education and training of PALS workers and acting as a resource for educational issues.

Concluding discussion: the way forward

The focus on inequalities is explicit, and the framework developed within the workstream has raised this as the priority for the work undertaken. Leicester Health Action Zone has been innovative in using education and training as a catalyst to address inequalities in health, and as is illustrated above this can then be 'integrated into mainstream activity' as stated as the main aim for HAZ in *Vision to reality* (DoH, 2001b).

A proposed externally funded evaluation of the workstream activities will be introduced, further illustrating the need to evaluate and identify priorities for future agendas, so central to HAZ at this time.

This chapter, and the work it reflects, is evidence that a well-structured approach to education and training can remain focused on the goal of reducing inequalities. The use of a framework that clearly prioritises addressing inequalities and service-user involvement can act as a catalyst to change services to better match the needs of the community.

The advantages of an affiliation to HAZ are clear: the Health Action Zone is impartial, as it is a virtual organisation or collection of partners. This creates at the same time a sense of impartiality that goes beyond the previous competitive internal market within the health service, and creates willingness for collaboration. The variety of partners within the HAZ opens doors to diverse ways of working across traditional organisational divides, e.g. the homeless and an education provider. It is unlikely that within the present climate any one of the partners could fulfil this role in isolation, underscoring the need for interdisciplinary inter-agency approaches for sustainable change.

Acknowledgement

The role of education and training within Leicester HAZ was initiated by Dr Angela Lennox, MBE, who continues as the workstream lead. Her tenacity and vision of the role and the potential of education and training as a catalyst for change and ameliorating inequalities underpin the activities reported here, and merit particular acknowledgement.

References

Balarajan, R. (1996) 'Ethnicity and variations in mortality from coronary heart disease', *Health Trends*, 28, 45–51.

DoH (1999) *National service framework for mental health: modern standards and service models*, London: Department of Health.

DoH (2000) *The NHS Plan: a plan for investment, a plan for reform*, London: Department of Health.

DoH (2001a) *Sexual health strategy*, London: Department of Health.

DoH (2001b) *Vision to reality*, London: Department of Health.

DoH (2001c) *Learning from Bristol: the report of the public inquiry into children's heart surgery at the Bristol Royal Infirmary, 1984–1995*, Cm 5207, London: Department of Health.

DoH (2001d) *The expert patient*, London: Department of Health.

HAZnet (2001) *Background: what are Health Action Zones?*, Health Development Agency [http://www.haznet.org.uk/hazs/background/background.asp].

Leicestershire Health Authority (2001) *Addressing health inequalities in Leicester, Leicestershire and Rutland: the annual report of the director of public health*, 11 May, Leicester: Leicestershire Health Authority.

OPCS (1991) *Census*, London: Office of Population Census and Surveys.

Sainsbury Centre for Mental Health (1997) *Pulling together: the future roles and training of mental health staff*, London: Sainsbury Centre.

Sainsbury Centre for Mental Health (2000) *The capable practitioner*, London: Sainsbury Centre.

Achievements, challenges and opportunities

Linda Bauld and Ken Judge

Health Action Zones were created at a time of when there was a great rebirth of enthusiasm for promoting public health. Since then there has been considerable policy turbulence as efforts to tackle health inequalities have been required to co-exist with wider efforts to modernise the delivery of public services in general and health care in particular. During the past five years policymakers and practitioners have experimented with numerous financial and institutional mechanisms in a search for the optimum form of health care organisation. As a result Health Action Zones have faced many challenges as they have tried to pursue their capacity building and health change goals. But despite, or perhaps even because of, the pressures that they have faced HAZs have made and are making considerable progress on a number of fronts. As a result, and as many of the contributions in this book have demonstrated, they have a major contribution to make to helping new organisations and their key personnel to learn from recent experience in such areas as partnership working, community involvement and tackling health inequalities. The aim of this brief concluding chapter is to set out in more general terms some of the important lessons to emerge from HAZs and to outline some of the key challenges and opportunities that remain.

We do this in three ways. Firstly, we summarise strategic lessons emerging from the national evaluation and HAZs themselves. Secondly, we outline the changing context in which HAZs are currently operating. Finally, we review how HAZs are responding to these changes and offer some final thoughts regarding the future.

Strategic lessons from the field

In addition to the evidence from local evaluation presented in the chapters of this volume, two recent outputs from the national evaluation and a report from the London and Luton HAZs provide examples of strategic lessons from the field. Interviews with HAZ project managers across all 26 Zones in November

2001, provide the first piece of evidence, and illustrate how HAZ principles are being translated into practice. After which some more detailed lessons emerging from two separate reports based on selected HAZs are outlined.

HAZ principles into practice

In November 2001, all 26 HAZ project managers were interviewed as part of the monitoring module of the national evaluation. They were asked to revisit the seven underlying principles of the initiative (shown in Box 1) and comment on the progress that had been made (Mackinnon et al, 2001).

Box 1: Underpinning principles of Health Action Zones

1. Achieving equity

Reducing health inequalities, promoting equality of access to services and improving equity in resource allocation

2. Engaging communities

Involving the public in planning services and empowering service users and patients to take responsibility for their own health and decisions about care

3. Working in partnership

Recognising that people receive services from a range of different agencies and that these services need to be co-ordinated to achieve the maximum benefit

4. Engaging front line staff

Involving staff in developing and implementing strategy, developing flexible and responsive organisations and encouraging and supporting innovation in service delivery

5. Taking an evidence-based approach

Having a more structured, evidence based approach for service planning and delivery as well as clinically effective procedures and interventions

6. Developing a person centred approach to service delivery

Developing services around the needs of people and delivering them as close to people as appropriate

7. Taking a whole systems approach

Recognising that health, social and other services are interdependent and need to be planned and organised on a whole system basis to deliver seamless care and tackle the wider determinants of health

---

Table 1 Perceived progress towards the seven HAZ principles

Principle	Mean	Minimum	Maximum
Achieving equity	2.6	1	4
Engaging communities	2.4	1	4
Working in partnership	1.7	1	3
Engaging frontline staff	2.9	2	5
Taking an evidence based approach	2.4	1	4
Developing a person centred approach to service delivery	2.3	1	4
Taking a whole systems approach	1.9	1	4

(Where 1 is 'excellent' and 5 is 'very poor', n = 26)

The responses that project managers provided in relation to the progress made towards each principle are illustrated in Table 1.

It is clear from these results that project managers assessed progress towards all of the seven principles relatively positively. 'Working in partnership' and 'taking a whole systems approach' accrued the highest scores, with 'engaging frontline staff' receiving the lowest score. One project manager felt that progress in engaging front line staff had been very poor. Five of the other principles also received at least one score of four, indicating relatively poor progress.

The aggregated mean for all seven principles was calculated for each of the HAZs to give an indication of overall progress across the 26. This is illustrated in Figure 1.

As Figure 1 illustrates, the general view expressed by project managers was that good progress had been made towards putting HAZ principles into practice. In explaining their responses, however, project managers did point out that

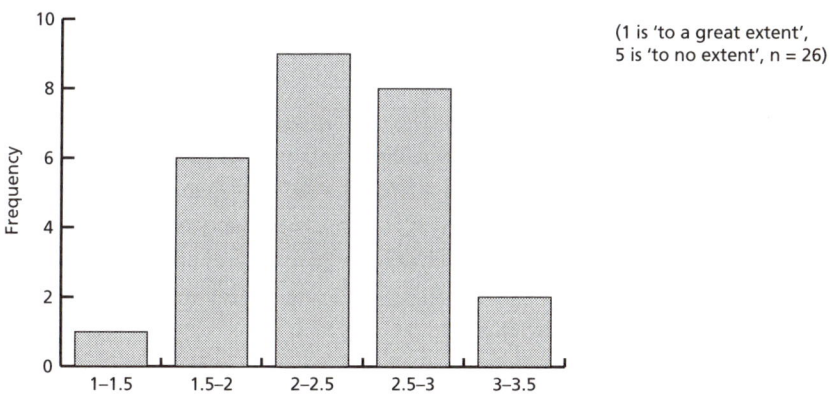

Figure 1: Aggregate mean scores for the seven underpinning principles of HAZ across all twenty-six zones

progress at this stage was in many cases more about putting issues on the agenda and establishing systems and frameworks than actually realising measurable change. In relation to 'achieving equity', for instance, the general feeling was that it was just too early to assess the contribution that HAZs had made, particularly in relation to health inequalities. Instead, project managers were more confident that the HAZ had contributed to raising awareness about inequalities and mechanisms for tackling them in the longer term. Similarly in relation to community involvement, project managers felt that infrastructures and mindsets had been changed, and that this would facilitate further progress.

Project managers also provided a range of examples of specific successes achieved by the HAZ. For the purposes of the interview and future evaluation fieldwork (that aims to examine examples of success in more detail), project managers were asked to list up to three successes. A wide range of examples were provided, most of which fell into one of the following categories:

- Projects or programmes focussing on specific groups, such as older people and children and young people
- Projects or programmes focussing on particular public health challenges, such as smoking, mental health and teenage pregnancy
- Projects or programmes addressing the determinants of health such as employment and housing
- Partnership structures and processes
- Community involvement and capacity building
- Modernisation, including service integration and work with secondary care
- Targeting and awareness raising regarding health inequalities
- Evaluation and learning processes or outputs
- Joining up with other initiatives
- Development of a HAZ/Resource directory

Project managers were also asked to provide information about the main areas in which their objectives had not been realised and further improvements were required. Again, given the huge range of activities that HAZs are involved in, the examples provided were very varied. But clear messages were available regarding the changes that need to be made if HAZs, and equally importantly their partner organisations, are to move towards addressing health inequalities in the future. Box 2 illustrates these changes.

Lessons from London and the Integrated Case Studies

Strategic lessons are also emerging from the eight HAZs that serve as integrated case studies (ICS) for the national evaluation. The first full year of ICS work is

Box 2: Areas of improvement needed in HAZs to help reduce inequalities

- Improved access to existing services and in the development of new services
- Improved educational attainment and lifelong learning
- More links between health and employment, income and poverty
- Improving the economic climate for the area and individuals
- Better partnership working and closer links with other initiatives
- Stronger public health leadership, particularly with ongoing structural changes in the NHS and local government
- Building capacity for tackling inequalities across all sectors and within the community

outlined in a recent report (Lawson et al, 2002). In addition, the four London HAZs and Luton HAZ have produced a summary of practical examples of how strategic learning has improved the way services are planned and delivered (MacDermott et al, 2002). Key themes include:

- Mechanisms for enabling change
- Balancing innovation and mainstreaming
- Support for learning
- HAZs and the wider reform agenda

Mechanisms for enabling change

In order to continue their work, HAZs like any other organisation or partnership need support and guidance from central government and adequate resources. In the introduction to this volume and in a number of other chapters, references have been made to the rapidly changing policy context that has made the process of HAZ development particularly fraught. The desire for commitment and clarity from the centre is a clear message emerging from the ICS work thus far. In particular, there is a need for (Lawson et al, 2002):

- Clarity about the key aims of the initiative – to date there have been inconsistent messages emerging from the centre regarding the purpose of HAZs – are they about responding to local needs, tackling the wider determinants of health or contributing to national policy priorities.

- Clarity about the timescale of the initiative – planning in the short term is different from planning for longer-term projects. HAZs were set up as a long term initiative yet funding decisions have been taken on a shorter term basis, meaning planning can only be done from year to year. If initiatives are to be short term, there need to be clear procedures in place to take forward learning so that best practice can move forward.
- Realistic objectives – even with a clear sense of direction realism about what can be achieved is still required. This has been a problem for HAZs, both centrally and locally.

The London and Luton HAZs also highlight the need for clarity and realistic timescales. They point to a number of prerequisites that need to be in place if change is to be achieved. This includes allowing a period of preparation and capacity-building to embed projects in the community. Skills, experience and resources need to be there before an initiative can begin its work (MacDermott et al, 2002). HAZs, like many other initiatives, have been victim to expectations of too much, too soon.

Other key mechanisms for change in HAZs have been building partnerships and engaging communities, as the chapters in the first section of this volume have highlighted. Effective partnership working requires engagement, commitment and investing in sustainable connections between organisations. Likewise, as the London/Luton HAZs point out, community involvement should pay attention to the aspirations of particular communities and not enforce collaboration inappropriately. They argue that building confidence will lead to long term integration and community cohesion.

Balancing innovation and mainstreaming

There is little doubt that HAZs have developed a range of innovative projects and ways of working. But there is an inherent tension between experimentation of this kind and longer-term changes in services. The London and Luton HAZs acknowledge this tension and argue that, based on their experience thus far, this can be resolved by supporting front line staff and communities to change the way services are developed and delivered. They highlight a number of key points (MacDermott et al, 2002, pg. 2):

- Frontline staff and communities need flexibility, time and money to influence strategy and service development
- Key frontline staff need to be identified as 'agents of change' and equipped with leadership and management skills.

- The service/team manager's role should be extended to include modernisation as well as operational tasks.
- Consistent leadership and a 'corporate' vision that is clearly communicated ensures that longer term change is possible, even when staff or priorities change.
- Champions of innovation are needed within partner agencies at a senior level.
- Recognition and validation of culturally specific and appropriate services for black and ethnic minority groups is required.
- Effective management is needed (although often neglected) both to plan major initiatives and individual projects.

The London and Luton HAZs also point to the need for 'developmental commissioning' to initiate innovative projects that then have a better chance of becoming part of mainstream projects. This involves replacing the competitive tendering process with a new system using facilitated partnerships and service level agreements.

Support for learning

Health Action Zones were intended to be learning organisations from their inception, as we outlined in the introduction to this volume. The emphasis on evidence-based practice and local and national evaluation has been consistent, but the relationship between investing in appropriate information gathering activities and transferring findings into practice has not always been clear. Support is required both to develop appropriate strategies and to use emerging evidence to demonstrate progress and to inform ongoing development.

In relation to strategy development, the ICS work has drawn attention to the fact that many of those involved in this activity within HAZs have had little or no prior experience and so require guidance and tools to assist them. The type of support needed is what is often described as 'technical assistance' from people with a range of relevant experience. To some extent this support for HAZs has come from the central DoH team and regional offices but there is little doubt that more input has been required in some areas. Realistic planning frameworks based on theories of change or log frame approaches have proved helpful in some instances. However, these frameworks are of limited utility without more sustained guidance regarding their use, and subsequent support to refine and modify strategies as programmes develop and emerging problems need to be resolved.

One barrier to successful strategy development and planning that the London and Luton HAZs identify is the lack of adequate baseline data to inform decisions. These HAZs and their partner organisations are investing in (MacDermott et al, 2002, pg. 4):

> ... the development of improved mapping of services to ensure a shared understanding of the local population so that all partners can work with the same baseline data. This has been most useful in identifying resource priorities and supporting funding bids. It is also useful for monitoring and evaluation purposes.

Shared and improved baseline information can facilitate the development of jointly agreed indicators and targets. This means that performance management frameworks can be shared between partner organisations. Demonstrating progress towards agreed objectives through the performance management process is a requirement for HAZs, but has been made considerably more difficult because of the lack of complementarity of information sources and systems between health and local authority, voluntary sector and other organisations. One of the achievements of HAZs has been investment in the development of joint frameworks, but more work of this kind is required.

Evaluation at the local level is another important source of information to demonstrate progress and inform ongoing development. There have been some tensions between the performance management process in HAZs and evaluation efforts. Evaluation should take a more in-depth approach than the monitoring required for performance management. But this has meant that expectations regarding what investment in evaluation will produce has often been unclear. Greater clarity regarding the relationship between national evaluation efforts, local evaluation and performance management has been called for from a number of HAZs. Even at this stage in their development, there is little consensus on the role of each and effective ways of reducing overlap. Newer initiatives such as New Deal for Communities (NDCs) are attempting to resolve this dilemma with clearer demarcation from the outset, supported by centrally generated guidelines, technical support and dissemination strategies.

This volume demonstrates the range of local evaluation efforts that HAZs are pursuing, and some early findings. These chapters represent just some of the evaluation work that is ongoing. Research and learning of this kind is central to the HAZ endeavour, but the extent to which it has and will influence developments across partner organisations and other initiatives remains to be seen. Effective support for and investment in local evaluation from the beginning is important, as is effective dissemination of findings. This book aims to contribute in part to dissemination, but it is equally important that a range of other types of information sharing take place at the local and national level.

HAZs and the wider reform agenda

Guaranteed funding for HAZs is currently not promised beyond March 2003. There is therefore a clear need to embed the achievements of HAZs to date in other emerging structures and programmes. Their contribution towards learning how to build effective partnerships to begin to address health inequalities needs to be captured and transferred. For this reason efforts are being made by individuals HAZs and within central government to forge links with new organisations such as Local Strategic Partnerships (LSPs) and Primary Care Trusts (PCTs), as well as build on relationships with other area-based initiatives such as Sure Start and NDCs. We turn now to examine this changing context, and the place of Health Action Zones within it.

The changing context

When HAZs were established, they inhabited a world populated with many institutions and policies that are now in the process of changing rapidly. In 1997/98 local authorities and health authorities were being encouraged to build partnerships to promote regeneration and health at a time when a plethora of area-based initiatives were jostling for position at the local level. Since then there has been a growing recognition of the need to develop a more coordinated approach to social change mechanisms at the local level. There have also been important moves in the direction of developing a more streamlined approach to service delivery not least in the NHS. To understand some of the challenges and opportunities now facing HAZs, it is important to understand some of these developments in relation to the reorganisation of the NHS and the new emphasis on neighbourhood renewal.

NHS reorganisation

The NHS in England is currently in the process of yet another major structural reorganisation (DoH, 2001). The main changes involve:

- giving PCTs new powers and control over resources to shape and commission services across the whole spectrum of hospital, community and primary services and from the whole range of possible providers in the public, private or voluntary sectors;
- leaving NHS Trusts with their current responsibilities whilst holding them to account through Strategic Health Authorities and requiring them to develop further patient and staff involvement in their own organisations and engage in creating networks for care with their partners externally;
- replacing health authorities by fewer and smaller Strategic Health Authorities with the responsibility for developing strategy and performance managing PCTs, NHS Trusts and Workforce Development Confederations so as to

secure delivery and consistency of approach. They will in effect manage the NHS on behalf of the Department of Health (DoH);

* reducing the DoH's direct role in management, abolishing its eight regional offices and creating 4 Directors of Health and Social Care to support and develop the NHS, provide local contact and performance manage the Strategic Health Authorities.

Strategic Health Authorities

Health Authorities are currently being merged into Strategic Health Authorities (StHAs), that will cover an average population of around 1.5m. While the responsibility for securing local health services will be devolved to PCTs, StHAs will provide strategic leadership to ensure the delivery of improvements in health and health services locally by PCTs and NHS Trusts within the national framework of developing a patient-centred NHS. The intention is that the wider span of control StHAs will have will enable them to consider the overall needs of the health economy across primary, community, secondary and tertiary care, and work with PCTs and NHS trusts to deliver a programme to meet these needs.

Primary Care Trusts

Primary Care Trusts (PCTs) are intended to be free-standing, statutory NHS bodies accountable to a Strategic Health Authority. PCTs have developed from Primary Care Groups, that were established following the abolition of GP Fundholding in 1997.

PCTs will take responsibility for securing the provision of the fuller range of services for the local populations, while StHAs step back from a hands-on commissioning role. PCTs will have responsibility for the management, development and integration of all primary care services including medical, dental, pharmaceutical and optical.

The size of the PCT will depend on the services it wishes to provide for its local population. PCTs will need to work in partnership with a range of other agencies outside the NHS to improve health and deliver wider objectives for social and economic regeneration. To facilitate this, they are also intended to be coterminous (either singly or jointly with another PCT) with a Local Authority boundary.

What this significant structural reform means for local communities is as yet unclear, but it currently involves a vast amount of upheaval in the health service that could temporarily affect the ability of some local health organisations to work effectively with other partners to promote population health and to reduce health inequalities. The *NHS Plan* specifically pledges that the NHS will play a key part in the implementation of key initiatives such as the *National Strategy for Neighbourhood Renewal*, but at the time of writing PCTs were still in the process of formation in some parts of the country, and front-line staff and managers in many parts of the health service are facing considerable uncertainty about the future.

The DoH is fully aware of the concerns and questions which have been raised about the reorganisation of the NHS, although it argues that these relate mainly to the detailed implementation of the proposals rather than the policy direction. A recent consultation exercise suggests that the main concerns expressed were about (DoH, 2002):

- the pace of change and concerns at the speed the DoH is moving (set against this, however, there is support from some NHS organisations for moving quickly);
- the capacity of PCTs to take on their new role fully from April 2002;
- scepticism as to whether or not they will have the adequate capability/capacity and resources to be robust organisations at the 'cornerstone' of the NHS;
- the disruption the changes may cause, and the ability of Health Authorities and subsequently Strategic Health Authorities to hold the programme together while they are re- organising and PCTs are developing.

It remains to be seen to what extent these difficulties are simply temporary ones or whether they hinder longer-term developments. But one thing does seem reasonably clear. If effective and sustainable change is to be brought about that enhances local commitment to promoting a comprehensive and modern public health agenda then Health Actions Zones have a vital role to play.

Neighbourhood Renewal

A New Commitment to Neighbourhood Renewal: A National Strategy Action Plan was launched by the Prime Minister at the beginning of 2001. The Strategy sets out the Government's vision for narrowing the gap between deprived neighbourhoods and the rest of the country, so that within a decade or so no citizen should be seriously disadvantaged by where they live. The aim is to deliver economic prosperity, safe communities, high quality education, decent housing, and better health to the poorest parts of the country. At the national level the Action Plan will be the responsibility of a new Neighbourhood Renewal Unit (NRU) located within the Department of Transport, Local Government and the Regions, which will be responsible for driving progress across Government (NRU, 2002).

To promote neighbourhood renewal, the Government has made a large number of promises to provide additional resources and to work in new and more co-ordinated and participative ways. Some of the key features of the approach include the following:

- Setting floor targets
- Providing additional resources
- Involving local communities and residents
- Strengthening Neighbourhood Management
- Improving Skills and Knowledge
- Learning from the New Deal for Communities programme
- Obtaining Better Information
- Developing Local Strategic Partnerships

Deprivation will be tackled through the bending of main Departmental programmes such as the police and health services, to focus more specifically on the most deprived areas. All relevant Departments now have minimum floor targets to meet, which are set out in Box 3.

Box 3 New floor targets

- Eliminate substandard social housing by 2010, and reduce it by a third by 2004;

- Ensure no area has burglary rates three times higher than the national average by 2005;

- Ensure at least 25% of pupils in every school and 38% in every local authority area achieve five or more GCSEs at grades A* to C;

- Starting with health authorities, by 2010 to reduce by at least 10 per cent the gap between the quintile of areas with the lowest life expectancy at birth and the population as a whole.

- Reduce, by at least 60 per cent by 2010, the conception rate among under 18s in the worst 20 per cent of wards, and thereby reduce the level of inequality between these areas and the average by at least 26 per cent by 2010.

- Raise employment in the 30 local districts with the worst labour market problems and narrow the gap between these and the overall rate.

A number of new funding streams have been made available to support the overall strategy. The Neighbourhood Renewal Fund, worth £900 million over 3 years, provides extra resources for 88 of the most deprived local authority districts. The Community Empowerment Fund of £36m over 3 years will support community and voluntary sector involvement in Local Strategic Partnerships in the 88 areas eligible for the Neighbourhood Renewal Fund (NRF). Neighbourhood Renewal Community Chests (£50m over 3 years) will provide small grants to formal and informal community groups to support community activity and mutual self-help in the 88 NRF areas. These grants are to be used in specific ways decided by local communities themselves, in conjunction with statutory and voluntary partner organisations. They are intended to help communities to take the first steps towards more formal involvement on their own terms.

The NRU is committed to ensuring a 'step change' in the level of skills and knowledge of everyone involved in neighbourhood renewal. To achieve this, there is a distinct skills and knowledge strand which runs throughout the Unit's work. This skills and knowledge element of neighbourhood renewal has two aims: to promote better sharing of knowledge about 'what works'; and to ensure that everyone involved in neighbourhood renewal has the skills to make a real difference.

The approach set out in the New Commitment to Neighbourhood Renewal is already being tried out on a smaller scale through the New Deal for Communities programme. NDC Partnerships have been established in 39 neighbourhoods across England. Over the ten-year duration of the programme they will receive funding totalling £1.9billion. Partnerships bring local communities together with mainstream service providers and other local stakeholders to tackle the problems in their neighbourhoods in an intensive and co-ordinated way.

Accurate information about social conditions is a powerful tool. It helps local and national partners to pinpoint problems and target solutions more effectively to renew the most deprived neighbourhoods. But such data at a neighbourhood level is not available - indeed lack of data means that many national targets for tackling deprivation are at the local authority level. The Neighbourhood Renewal Unit and the Office for National Statistics are developing better data on all aspects of deprivation at the neighbourhood level.

Neighbourhood Renewal at the local level will be the responsibility of the Local Strategic Partnership, which will bring together public, private and voluntary sector service providers with the community and business sectors (NRU, 2001). They will offer the opportunity to rationalise the many partnerships that exist already. This consolidation process is intended to include Health Action Zones.

Local Strategic Partnerships' core tasks are to:

- develop and deliver a local neighbourhood renewal strategy to secure more jobs, better education, improved health, reduced crime, and better housing, narrowing the gap between deprived neighbourhoods and the rest and contributing to the national targets to tackle deprivation.

- prepare and implement a community strategy for the area, identify and deliver the most important things which need to be done, keep track of progress, and keep it up-to-date;
- bring together local plans, partnerships and initiatives to provide a forum through which mainstream service providers (local authorities, the police, health services, central government agencies, and bodies outside the public sector and so on) work effectively together to meet local needs and priorities;
- work with local authorities that are developing a local public service agreement (PSA) to help devise and then meet suitable targets.

How are HAZs responding?

When key local actors in Health Action Zones were interviewed at the end of 2001, they were asked about the extent to which HAZs are linking with Local Strategic Partnerships and Primary Care Trusts. Project managers were asked to describe the level of involvement of their HAZ in LSP development. The results are summarised in Figure 2.

As Figure 2 shows, eighteen (69%) project managers perceive the role of their HAZ in LSP development to be 'leading' or 'significant'. In response to a subsequent question, nineteen (73%) project managers reported that their HAZ has very good or good relations with the (developing) PCTs in their area. Only two (8%) project managers felt this was true to a lesser extent. Relations with HAZs may be important for PCTs and LSPs as they are a potential source of knowledge, skills and learning. Project managers were also asked to what extent they

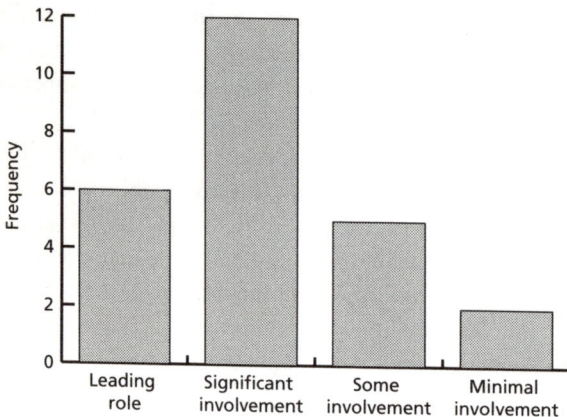

Figure 2: Level of involvement of HAZs in LSP development

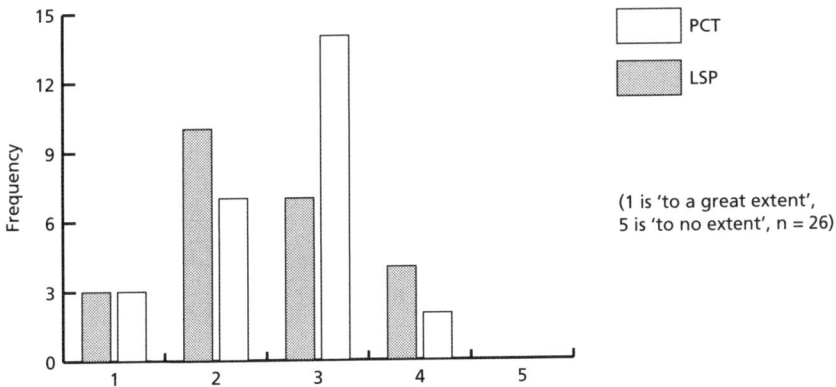

Figure 3: Extent to which project managers feel that learning from HAZs is being transferred to LSPs and PCTs

felt that learning from HAZs was being transferred to the LSP and PCTs. The results, which are shown in Figure 3, are quite promising, especially in relation to LSPs. But they also imply that more work needs to be done to exploit investments in learning by HAZs.

Our view is that it is vital that the capacity of LSPs and PCTs to learn from the work and experiences of HAZs should be maximised. A recent evaluation of the first wave of LSPs (New Commitment to Regeneration Phase 1 Pathfinders) outlines the importance of transferring learning from existing initiatives, such as HAZs, to LSPs (Russell, 2001). Unless adequate investment in this area is made, LSPs are at risk of 'reinventing the wheel', particularly in relation to building multi-agency partnerships and engaging communities. Project managers clearly believe that there is a real potential for HAZs to contribute to this learning, and are now investing considerable energy in building strong links with these emerging organisations.

A final word

Much of the work that HAZs have been undertaking in the past 3 or 4 years is now to be taken forward by PCTs and LSPs. Between them these two new organisational structures have key local responsibilities to promote public health and to tackle social exclusion and reduce health inequalities. The key continuing responsibility of HAZs in these circumstances is to help these new and relatively fragile organisations to meet the challenges that they face. The ways in which the 26 health action zones will do this varies from area to area. In some instances the HAZ is coterminous with a single PCT and ensuring continuity of purpose will be relatively straightforward. In other areas more complex arrangements are being put in place, but whatever the precise plans that are envisaged it will take some time before they are running smoothly. In the meantime everyone associated with HAZs should be encouraged to take the opportunity to use the knowledge and experienced gained in recent years to ensure that the hard won lessons learnt about promoting local public health strategies and modernising health care delivery systems are not lost. The main message from this book is that there is a rich vein of learning that can be drawn upon.

References

Department of Health (2001) *Shifting the Balance of Power within the NHS: Securing Delivery*. July 2001, http://www.doh.gov.uk/shiftingthebalance/initialconsult.htm

Department of Health (2002) *Shifting the Balance of Power: the next steps*. Annex A. January 2002. http://www.doh.gov.uk/shiftingthebalance/index.htm

Lawson, L., Mackenzie, M., Mackinnon, J., Meth, F., and Truman, J. (2002) *Health Action Zones Integrated Case Studies: Preliminary findings*, Health Promotion Policy Unit, University of Glasgow. Available at: http://www.haznet.org.uk

MacDermott, K., Nessling, B., Findaly, G, Dear, S., and Vernon, P (2002) *Investing Our Learning in the Future: key strategic learning from the London and Luton Health Action Zones*, Lambeth, Southwark and Lewisham HAZ, London.

Mackinnon, J., Bauld, L., Lawson, L., and Judge, K. (2001) *Monitoring Interviews: Autumn 2001 Summary Report*, Health Promotion Policy Unit, University of Glasgow, November 2001. Available at: http://www.haznet.org.uk

Neighbourhood Renewal Unit (2001) *Local Strategic Partnerships*. Department of, Transport, Local Government and the Regions, October 2001. http://www.neighbourhood.dtlr.gov.uk/overview/index.htm

Neighbourhood Renewal Unit (2002) *The Vision for Neighbourhood Renewal*. Department of Transport, Local Government and Regions. January 2002. http://www.neighbourhood.dtlr.gov.uk/overview.index.htm

Russell, H. (2001) – *Local Strategic Partnerships. Lessons from New Commitment to Regeneration*, Area Regeneration Series, The Policy Press, Bristol.

Index